QUESTIONS
from the
HEART

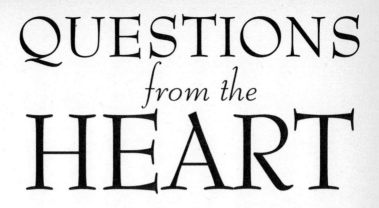

QUESTIONS
from the
HEART

*Answers to 100 Questions About
Chelation Therapy, a Safe Alternative
to Bypass Surgery*

TERRY CHAPPELL, M.D.
PREFACE BY JULIAN WHITAKER, M.D.

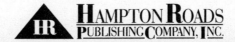

HAMPTON ROADS
PUBLISHING COMPANY, INC.

Cover design by Matthew Friedman

For information write:

Hampton Roads Publishing Company, Inc.
134 Burgess Lane
Charlottesville, VA 22902

Or call: (804) 296-2772
FAX: (804) 296-5096

If you are unable to order this book from your local
bookseller, you may order directly from the publisher.
Quantity discounts for organizations are available.
Call 1-800-766-8009, toll-free.

ISBN 1-57174-026-0

10 9 8 7 6 5 4 3

Printed in Canada

Table of Contents

Foreword

Another Way
by Philip O'Connor

It's an old story. A man, usually in his mid-fifties, develops suspicious symptoms—chest pains, shortness of breath, or maybe only skipped heart beats—and reports them to his family physician. The doctor tells him that the symptoms may not amount to anything serious but that, to be safe, the patient ought to have an electrocardiogram. The patient nervously agrees. (Is there really any choice?) The next day he undergoes the routine and painless test. The doctor lets him know almost immediately afterwards that the results are negative. "But," the doctor adds, "because of your age, let's not take any chances. I'd like you to have an exercise stress test." The patient soon learns that the stress test will measure heart function not at rest but during activities that accurately mirror fairly vigorous activity. "I'm not worried," the doctor says.

"Why should *he* be?" thinks the patient. "It's *my* ticker they're going to be checking out."

The following day the patient reports to the local hospital, where another doctor, a stranger, oversees the patient's workout on the treadmill. After about two minutes the patient experiences a slight shortness of breath, the same shortness of breath he's now and then experienced when he's taken the family dog for a morning stroll. Now, however, he can't stop and let his breath catch up. He must keep walking on a surface that increasingly steepens. "No problem," he tells himself. The chest pain is, after all, mild and not getting more severe.

"Stop the test," the anonymous doctor says suddenly to the nurse or technician who had earlier taped the electrodes to the man's chest and is now monitoring the treadmill machine. Immediately the patient feels the treadmill stop.

"What's wrong?" he says. "I could have kept going."

He's not helped by the anonymous doctor's response: "Your family doctor will give you a full report."

"Well," says the family doctor lightheartedly after calling his patient the following day. "It looks as though we're going to have to keep letting you get your money's worth out of that insurance company of yours." The doctor explains that the stress test indicated "possible heart disease," but quickly adds that simple exercise stress tests are not always accurate. "I'd like you to see the cardiologist I work with." The patient is alarmed by the mention of heart disease and is not at all comforted by the news that it's not yet real, only "possible."

"Just to be safe?" he says.

"That's right," his family physician replies in a reassuring tone. "Just to be safe."

The cardiologist is a young man, perhaps twenty years younger than the patient. He says that his father is a family physician who says that his son is only "a vest pocket doctor." He smiles and points to his chest, in case the patient missed the joke. After a friendly chat the cardiologist has the patient take an in-office echogram, which, he's informed the patient, will provide a good look at the chambers of the heart. Just minutes after the test is completed, the cardiologist tells the patient he's seen nothing unusual but adds, matter-of-factly, that he'd like to have a closer look at the condition of the patient's arteries by having him take a thallium stress test. This time, while on the treadmill, the patient will be injected with radioactive thallium, which will enable the doctor to determine, among other things, whether there has been damage as a result of a previous heart attack. "That first stress test was inconclusive," the physician says. "I'll feel more comfortable looking at this more complete test."

Another anonymous doctor, this one at the cardiologist's big city hospital, lets the patient stay on the treadmill for five minutes, nearly two more minutes than he was allowed to last during the first test. "A good sign," the patient thinks as he lies still while a big x-ray machine records the post-test activity of the thallium. The patient is still thinking optimistically the next day when he returns to the cardiologist's office to get the final results of the testing.

"I'm sorry," says the cardiologist, "but we're just going to have to get a closer look at that heart of yours. The thallium test indicated that you might have some pretty large blockages in at least two of your arteries." There is no joking now, no light-heartedness. "I want you to have an angiogram in the next few days. Let's see how bad it is." He is soon sharing the bad news with his wife, telling her that the angiogram will show just where the blockages are. "Then what?" she says.

"I may have to have to have coronary artery bypass surgery."

Until now, the patient has felt he had no choice but to go to the next step. Now, frightened by the prospect of an invasion of his body with wires and tubes and later a saw and other unpleasant instruments, he takes counsel with himself. He remembers his old high-school buddy, who had a bypass operation a few years ago and had to go back for another just a year ago. He recalls the article on alternative medicine he read in the "Living" section of the Sunday paper. One of the alternative methods discussed was EDTA Chelation Therapy. Somewhere he's saved that article. He decides to dig it out and get the name of the chelation physician who was interviewed. "There may be another way," he tells his wife.

The patient believes in God, country, apple pie, and the efficacy of standard medicine. He therefore feels guilty when he decides to look into other ways of dealing with his heart disease. He nevertheless makes his way to the city's main health food store where the owner and manager mentions EDTA Chelation Therapy and introduces him to two books on the subject, Dr. Elmer Cranton's *Bypassing Bypass* and Dr. Morton Walker's *The Chelation Way*. The owner tells him about several customers who, for one reason or another, all suffering from heart disease, chose EDTA Chelation Therapy over bypass surgery. "They're all doing very well," he says. Why, then, the patient wants to know, don't physicians recommend chelation therapy instead of bypass surgery? "Read those books, and others on the subject," says the owner.

The patient goes home and begins reading and is soon persuaded that EDTA Chelation Therapy deserves consideration. At the health food store library he finds Arline Brecher's book, *Forty-Something Forever,* where he reads about a man who asked his insurance company (a major one) to pay for his chelation therapy. The company refused, and the man took his case to the courts. The case was heard by Judge George H. Ferguson, who declared:

> Although chelation therapy may not be the treatment of choice for atherosclerosis, it appears to be a broadly accepted professional treatment since 300,000 patients have received intravenous EDTA chelation treatments over the past thirty years and with fewer than twenty deaths compared to more than four thousand deaths caused by coronary artery bypass surgery in approximately an equal number of cases.

Our patient's research is interrupted by a phone call from the cardiologist's nurse, who says the doctor would like to go ahead and schedule bypass surgery the following week. The patient remembers the cardiologist telling him "There's really no time to waste. Quite frankly, you could drop dead at any moment." The patient feels a tightness in his chest, the first in days and takes it as evidence that the cardiologist is right. Yet, for some reason—"a gut reason," he will tell his wife later—he asks the nurse not to schedule anything yet. "I'll get back to you soon," he promises.

For the first time he pops into his mouth one of the nitroglycerine tablets the cardiologist gave him earlier. When the tightness in his chest subsides, he picks up his phone and calls the nutrition store. "I'd like to consult with a chelation doctor," he tells the owner. "Can you recommend one?" The health store owner gives him the names and phone numbers of an M.D. and two osteopathic doctors who practice chelation therapy. He calls the M.D. and makes an appointment.

The atmosphere in the chelation doctor's office is strikingly different than the somber silence of the cardiologist's waiting room or even the finger-tapping uneasiness in the crowded waiting area of the patient's family doctor. Here people are speaking to each other, sharing information about their diets, boasting about their improved conditions. Is the patient imagining the happy atmosphere?

Until now, we haven't given him a name for, in fact, he has been one of those nameless trusting people who, for whatever reason, follow commonly prescribed ways in almost all aspects of their lives. Only now is he making a striking exception, in effect saying that he will take control of his own health, no matter what, including the criticism and doubts of others, even his friends and family. He is frightened but feels somehow right about his decision.

Bob is soon in the chelation doctor's office introducing himself. "I'm Bob Powers," he says, "and I'm looking into the possibility of having chelation therapy." Dr. Edward Church is a tranquil man, about forty, who listens with a curious, interested expression as Bob recounts all that has happened since he first reported his heart condition to his family physician.

"I'm curious about chelation, but frightened too," Bob says. "And I have a hundred questions."

The doctor nods. "We welcome questions," he says, and for the next twenty minutes answers the most pressing questions his new patient offers.

Like Bob Powers, I was told by a standard cardiologist two years ago that I had major blockages in all of the arteries around my heart. Like Bob, I explored EDTA Chelation Therapy as an alternative to bypass surgery. I began treatments, as Bob did, shortly after my first meeting with my chelation doctor, L. Terry Chappell, M.D. I have had nearly fifty injections, and they have certainly been successful. The symptoms that caused me to contact Dr. Chappell have completely vanished. The cost of my treatments, tests, and vitamin and mineral supplements have been about $8,500. That is certainly much less than the $120,000 a friend, who has had bypass surgery, estimates he has cost his insurance company. (And he still has many of the symptoms that brought him to a cardiologist to begin with!) I have also had chelation treatments, while traveling, from Dr. Paul Lynn, M.D., in San Francisco, and David Edwards, M.D., in Reno. All of these doctors are well-informed, patient-oriented, and more willing to answer questions than time permits.

I suggested to Dr. Chappell that he answer, in book form, a series of questions, based on real questions asked by people contemplating undergoing EDTA Chelation Therapy. He agreed to do this, and the work that follows is the result.

Preface

by Julian Whitaker, M.D.

In the United States in 1991, $10 billion dollars was spent on bypass surgery for heart disease that, according to the best medical literature available, is no better than a handful of heart pills taken every day.

And yet Chelation Therapy, an outpatient (office) procedure which can restore normal vascular and cellular function with extreme safety and effectiveness has been largely suppressed by those who make medical policy decisions and control the economic purse strings of medical insurance companies.

I have documented 10 points showing that most bypass surgery is a total waste of money. The evidence for these points comes from the most prestigious medical journals in the world.

1. The *best* that can be said about bypass and balloon angioplasty is that they are irrelevant to the natural course of the disease (with a few important exceptions). Patients treated medically with drugs live just as long and just as well. The worst that can be said for this approach is that the procedures are a terrible hoax, increasing disability, suffering, and death among hundreds of thousands of trusting heart patients.

2. Cardiac catheterization is an inaccurate method to determine what is going on with the disease. There is great and unpredictable variability in interpretation of the same x-rays from one radiologist to the next and even with the same radiologist, if the same films are shown to him at different times.

3. The angiogram is so inaccurate that it is not even a reliable estimate of blood flow restriction. That is, a 90-percent blockage has been shown to have more brisk blood flow than a blockage read as 40 percent.

4. The cardiopulmonary pump used during bypass surgery may cause decreased oxygen to the brain while in operation and thus often leads to brain damage, memory loss, and personality changes postoperatively.

5. The number of vessels blocked should be irrelevant to the need for bypass surgery. The main factor of significance is how well the left ventricular pump is working. Bypass appears helpful only in the narrow window of an ejection fraction of only 30 to 40 percent.

6. One hundred fifty people who refused bypass, according to one study, did far better than would have been expected had the surgery been done.

7. After grafting, the rate of plaque formation in the "upstream" segment of the grafted artery is ten times the rate confirmed in an intact coronary artery. The upstream closure starves the heart upstream.

8. After a bypass operation, the incidence of a subsequent heart attack or myocardial infarction occurring is higher than with those treated medically. This is especially true of silent MI's, which may be just as dangerous but do not present significant chest pain.

9. Up to 90 percent of bypass procedures are done when the ejection fraction (or pump function) is greater than 50 percent, which is adequate for the heart to do its job, and indicates an excellent prognosis without surgery.

10. In patients over 80 years of age, 25 to 33 percent of them die within one year of bypass surgery. This is an incredibly high mortality rate that is far greater than with medical therapy.

In contrast, according to the American College for Advancement in Medicine, more than 500,000 patients have received therapy with intravenous EDTA Chelation Therapy under the modern protocol that was adopted almost twenty years ago, and no deaths have been reported that were directly attributable to use of this protocol.

Many studies, both published and unpublished, have established the efficacy rate at about 85% in patients treated with chelation. Since circulation improves all over the body with chelation, there are many beneficial "side effects" and only a few adverse ones.

Chelation Therapy, the process of injecting a drug with metal binding properties for the reduction of toxic metals, dates back to 1950 in the United States.

Workers suffering from lead intoxication in a battery factory were treated with ethylene diamine tetraacetic acid (EDTA). In addition to lead, EDTA also binds with iron, copper, and calcium. Coincidentally, it was noted that patients treated for lead poisoning who also had coronary artery disease improved in that realm as well.

With the advent of heart surgery and many new vascular drugs, scientific interest waned. A small group of complementary physicians continued to use the therapy through the '70s and '80s.

Recent research studies again document dramatic improvement. A retrospective study of Chelation Therapy using EDTA (Olszewer and Carter 1988) that included 2,850 patients showed significant improvement in patients with peripheral vascular disease and ischemic heart disease. This was accompanied by numerous smaller studies, many of them by McDonagh, Rudolph and Cheraskin and a large as-yet-unpublished study of 19,000 patients showing about 85 percent of the treated group with measurable improvement in their vascular status. The only negative clinical study to date was done by a group of vascular surgeons from Denmark, and an editorial in the *Journal for Advancement in Medicine* has claimed that study to be seriously flawed, if not fraudulent.

Another group of Danish doctors chelated 65 patients who were on the waiting list for bypass surgery and 58 of them were able to cancel their surgery. The time for wide acceptance of EDTA Chelation Therapy will soon be here.

Dr. Terry Chappell has provided us with an excellent book, answering the important questions that all cardiovascular patients and others at risk need to have answered about Chelation Therapy.

Julian Whitaker
June 1995

References for Dr. Whitaker's comments may be found at the end of the book.

Introduction

Knowing the truth about the results of using EDTA Chelation Therapy as a treatment for vascular disease may save your life or the life of someone you love. Every year in the United States we spend $10,000,000,000 on a medical procedure—bypass surgery—that in many cases is unnecessary.

Every year more people in our country die of complications from taking prescription medications exactly as directed than are killed in auto accidents. Yet we have another medical procedure, called Chelation Therapy, which utilizes a more natural approach to restore normal vascular and cellular function. This procedure has been largely suppressed, and there are many misconceptions about the therapy.

Questions have remained on this controversial subject. With the considerable help of well-known author Philip O'Connor of Bowling Green University, who was undergoing Chelation Therapy for his coronary artery disease at my office, I decided it would be helpful to ask all of my chelation patients what questions they most wanted answered regarding their therapy.

The questions were compiled, and I have tried to provide the answers. Rather than arrange the questions in a particular order, I have arranged them as they may have been asked at one of the many seminars I have given on the subject. For your convenience in searching for a specific topic, the questions are listed in the first section, which follows..

Appendices I and II include the texts of the two meta-analyses (study of studies) that I wrote with Dr. John Stahl, showing scientific evidence on the effectiveness of EDTA treatment of cardiovascular disease.

Appendices III and IV are two bibliographies, the first documenting the startling observations of Dr. Julian Whitaker about the terrible misuse of bypass surgery in the United States in recent years, and the second providing references on the mechanism of action of EDTA Chelation Therapy for arterio-sclerotic cardiovascular disease.

The more we understand about this revolutionary treatment for the number-one killer disease in the United States, the better off we will be. Read the book and give it to your friends and loved ones. If you choose to become a patient of one the courageous, knowledgeable doctors who offer EDTA Chelation as a treatment option, the book will help you cooperate with your doctor and enhance the effects of your therapy.

The Questions
and Where to Find the Answers

#1 What is Chelation Therapy? (p. 29)

#2 Can you describe how this works to improve blood flow to the heart? (p. 30)

#3 Coronary artery bypass surgery is the standard American Medical Association approved method for improving circulation to the heart. Why should a person consider chelation therapy, and choose it when he or she has been diagnosed and found to have substantial blockages of the coronary arteries? (p. 30)

#4 Is there any case of atherosclerosis or arteriosclerosis where you would recommend Coronary Artery Bypass Graft Surgery over Chelation Therapy? (p. 32)

#5 Many notable persons, such as Henry Kissinger and Alexander Haig, had CABG more than ten years ago and seem to be doing well. How do you explain this, and can similar or better results be obtained from Chelation Therapy? (p. 33)

#6 How do the complications following CABG compare with those following Chelation Therapy? (p. 33)

#7 What do surgeons say to convince patients to submit to bypass surgery? (p. 34)

#8 In recent years, numerous other alternatives to Coronary Artery Bypass Graft Surgery have been used experimentally—such as laser surgery, rotoectomy, and a combination of diet, yoga, and exercise. How do the results of these compare with results from Chelation Therapy? (p. 35)

#9 If chelation is so good, why isn't everyone using it? (p. 36)

#10 There is a general public ignorance about Chelation Therapy as a treatment for CABG. Can you explain this? (p. 36)

#11 Why did the FDA raid the office of Dr. Jonathan Wright? Are you afraid of a similar raid? (p. 37)

#12 How about medical board sanctions? (p. 37)

#13 Why such a detailed "informed consent"? (p. 38)

#14 What objections do the AMA and other conventional medical organizations have against Chelation Therapy? (p. 38)

#15 What are the current costs of CABG and Chelation Therapy, including long-range maintenance? (p. 40)

#16 Why are supplemental vitamins, minerals, and herbs used in conjunction with Chelation Therapy? (p. 41)

#17 How is diet used to supplement Chelation Therapy? (p. 42)

#18 Why are Chelation Therapy treatments given once or twice a week? Why do they take 3 to 4 hours to be completed? (p. 42)

#19 What percentage of patients are improved after Chelation Therapy? (p. 43)

#20 Why do the remaining 10 to 15 percent not receive similar benefits? (p. 43)

#33 Can you give specific examples of efforts made by chelation physicians to have such studies made? (p. 49)

#34 Is there currently a study comparing Chelation Therapy to CABG at numerous Veterans Hospitals? (p. 50)

#35 Surely some preliminary results have been reported. If so, what do they indicate? (p. 50)

#36 Are there other studies, not considered anecdotal, that can be used to make the case for Chelation Therapy over CABG? (p. 51)

#37 About what percentage of your patients have come to you as a result of failed CABG? (p. 51)

#38 Can you describe a typical case? (p. 52)

#39 What have been the results both long-range and short-range of this patient? (p. 53)

#40 What part does mental attitude play with Chelation Therapy? (p. 53)

#41 What kind of water should I drink? Is distilled water important? (p. 53)

#42 Why is distilled water recommended over spring water or purified water like that available in supermarkets? (p. 54)

#43 If I am traveling while undergoing chelation treatments, can I continue treatments elsewhere? (p. 55)

#44 How can I find a reputable chelation doctor who will continue my treatments? (p. 55)

#45 How can I be sure that the treatments I am getting in another location are the same as those I receive from you? (p. 55)

#46 Can you cite patients who have completed an initial chelation therapy (the full cycle) and who are willing to testify to the effectiveness of their treatment? (p. 56)

#47 What goes on at the meetings of the American College for Advancement in Medicine (ACAM) and the Great Lakes Association for Clinical Medicine (GLACM)? (p. 56)

#48 If you yourself suffered chest pains with a related diagnosis of atherosclerosis, would you take the same treatments you recommend to others? (p. 57)

#49 What can a convinced layman do to help open the eyes of those who have been blind to the beneficial effects of Chelation Therapy? (p. 57)

#50 What are the most common side effects, if any, of Chelation Therapy? (p. 58)

#51 What are some of the aftereffects of Chelation? (p. 59)

#52 What causes the delayed improvement that you sometimes see after a patient has completed a course of chelation therapy? (p. 59)

#53 What do you think of oral chelation? Is it as effective as I.V. Chelation Therapy? (p. 60)

#54 Can oral chelation be used as maintenance? (p. 60)

#55 Can oral chelation be used between regular weekly chelation treatments? (p. 60)

#56 Have you ever given up on a coronary artery patient and recommend that he or she submit themselves for CABG surgery? (p. 61)

#57 Describe a worst-case scenario and how you would treat it. (p. 61)

#58 Some people recommend a low-carbohydrate diet and others recommend a high-carbohydrate diet, but with a reduction in refined sugars. How do I know which one works best and which one I should use? (p. 61)

#59 After I start EDTA treatments, when can I increase my activity? (p. 63)

#60 Should my medicines be reduced when taking chelation therapy? (p. 63)

#61 Can I get off all my medications? (p. 63)

#62 If my I.V. hurts at the place where the needle is in my arm, what can be done? (p. 64)

#63 I hate to take so many pills! Are they all necessary? (p. 64)

#64 My family history is bad for heart disease but I seem to be healthy. Should I take chelation as a prevention treatment? (p. 64)

#65 Is caffeine a problem? (p. 65)

#66 Should I take aspirin along with my chelation treatments? (p. 65)

#67 Should I take vitamin E? (p. 65)

#68 How about fish oils? (p. 66)

#69 When is a patient too old to take chelation therapy? (p. 66)

#70 Will it help Alzheimer's Disease? (p. 66)

#71 Will chelation help arthritis? (p. 67)

#72 Will chelation help Parkinson's Disease? (p. 67)

#86 Can Chelation Therapy help an aneurysm? (p. 74)

#87 Should milk be consumed while a patient is taking chelation therapy? (p. 75)

#88 Is it possible that women who are taking calcium supplements to prevent osteoporosis could be contributing to their heart attacks and strokes? (p. 75)

#89 Does EDTA have some side benefits that may treat cancer or arthritis? (p. 76)

#90 Why does my angina come and go? (p. 76)

#91 Why are recliner chairs used? (p. 77)

#92 Define "saw-tooth" progress. (p. 77)

#93 Does EDTA help varicose veins? (p. 77)

#94 What determines the cost of the I.V.? (p. 78)

#95 Why can't chelation be given at home? (p. 78)

#96 How about patient support groups? (p. 78)

#97 What can I do if I cannot afford Chelation Therapy? (p. 79)

#98 If I can't change to a perfect lifestyle, am I wasting my money in taking chelation? (p. 79)

#99 How do I find heavy metal toxicity and can I use that for a diagnosis? (p. 80)

#100 If I have an excess amount of heavy metals in my urine, will insurance pay for my treatment? (p. 80)

Dr. Chappell Answers
Your Questions
about
Chelation Therapy

#1 What is Chelation Therapy?

Chelation is derived from the Greek word meaning "claw." In chemical terms it means to surround and take with. EDTA is the most common medicine used for Chelation Therapy. It is a synthetic amino acid that removes toxic metals, such as lead, cadmium, aluminum, and arsenic. It also lowers the level of calcium from the bloodstream as well as excessive iron and copper. The net effect of these actions are as follows:

1. It serves as an antioxidant. Too much oxidation causes deterioration all over the body, much like hard water causes accumulation of metal deposits on the walls of pipes.

2. It serves as an anticoagulant, so that the blood doesn't clot as easily.

3. It is a potent reducer of calcium in the blood stream and subsequently in soft tissue. This reduces the hard part of the hardening of the arteries, as well as stiffening in the tissues.

4. At the cell membrane, it stabilizes lipid peroxidation, which is a chemical breakdown of fats that interferes with the action of all cells in the body. It does this by removing iron and copper which increase the chemical process.

5. It causes magnesium to move into the cell to replace calcium that has been removed. This makes for a much healthier cell that is less likely to go into spasm.

6. By removing the toxic metals, it reduces the atherogenic process of laying down plaque in the vessels which is stimulated by these metals.

(29)

7. It reduces blood pressure by reducing spasm of the vessels and by the removal of lead.

By these mechanisms of action, EDTA improves circulation throughout the body in both large and small vessels, and also improves cell-membrane function in all the tissues of the body. I have listed almost forty references about these mechanisms in the Bibliography.

#2 Can you describe how this works to improve blood flow to the heart?

Normal heart function is dependent on good perfusion of the coronary arteries, which supply nutrients and oxygen to the heart. Reduced coronary blood flow is due either to the development of plaque, which obstructs the flow to the heart, or the spasm of the muscles in the coronary arteries, which also reduces the blood flow. EDTA will reduce the plaque to a certain extent, and it will make the blood vessels softer and more flexible so that more blood can get through. By improving cell-membrane function it also reduces the tendency toward decreased blood flow from spasm that can result in angina pectoris, or chest pain.

#3 Coronary artery bypass surgery is the standard American Medical Association approved method for improving circulation to the heart. Why should a person consider Chelation Therapy, and choose it when he or she has been diagnosed and found to have substantial blockages of the coronary arteries?

It is true CABG (Coronary Artery Bypass Graft Surgery) is the standard therapy in the United States. There were 80,000 operations performed in 1976; 200,000 in 1985; and about 500,000 in 1992.

However, there is mounting evidence in the literature that CABG operations are no more effective than standard medical therapy. Henry MacIntosh, who is a cardiologist at Baylor

College of Medicine and a colleague of the famed heart surgeon Dr. Michael DeBakey, reviewed all the cases they had operated on over a ten-year period. His paper had 220 references, and his conclusions were as follows:

1. There is symptomatic improvement, but this does not persist;

2. Cardiac arrhythmias and congestive heart failure are not prevented by CABG; and

3. Life is *not* prolonged by CABG.

A large Veteran's Administration Hospital study showed that after three years of therapy, 87 percent of the medically treated group were alive and 88 percent of the surgically treated group were alive. There was no significant difference between the two groups. The CASS Study was a large study performed by the country's best cardiovascular surgeons from Stanford, the Cleveland Clinic, and other prestigious centers. The study compared the medically and the surgically treated groups over a ten-year period and showed:

1. The operation does not relieve pain; and

2. There were no significant differences in the employment or recreational status of the patients.

Even with triple vessel disease, the annual mortality rate is no more than 2 percent per year, whereas the operative mortality rate for CABG surgery is approximately 5 percent on the table and there is a similar mortality to medical therapy each year.

Another common therapy is balloon angioplasty, which dilates isolated blockages in selected coronary arteries. Unfortunately, the results from this procedure are not any better. According to a *Medical Tribune* article in May 1993, 50 percent of angioplasties have to be repeated within six months and the death rate following angioplasty for coronary artery disease is also 2 percent per year, or one out of every 50 people.

Dr. Thomas Graboys of Harvard heads up a clinic that gives second opinions for cardiovascular problems. He has published the results which show that approximately 70 percent of people who come to his clinic with bypass surgery recommended do not need the procedure. Even further, approximately 80 percent of those who have had catheterization recommended to study the coronary arteries do not even need to have the cath!

In contrast, there is increasing evidence that Chelation Therapy *improves* circulation in a large majority of patients and significantly improves the quality of life.

A recent meta-analysis (study of studies), which Dr. John Stahl of Ohio Northern University and I conducted, collected 40 published studies and another 30 which have not yet been published. These studies were from the United States and six other countries. All together the studies looked at almost 25,000 patients treated with EDTA chelation for vascular disease. All but one of the multi-patient studies, which was done by a group of Danish cardiac surgeons (on patients who, for the most part, continued to smoke), showed positive results. Eighty-seven percent of the patients had measurable improvement in their vascular disease. The paper describing the published studies on chelation is included at the end of this book in its entirety.

#4 Is there any case of atherosclerosis or arteriosclerosis where you would recommend Coronary Artery Bypass Graft Surgery over Chelation Therapy?

Yes, indeed! There are a few patients, whose left ventricular function (which is responsible for propelling the blood to all of the body except the lungs) is between 25 and 50 percent of what it should be, and who do not respond to Chelation Therapy or medications, who have a high probability that they would benefit from Coronary Artery Bypass Graft Surgery. Those patients are not commonly found, and if they do require the surgery, I would recommend that they receive Chelation Therapy afterwards.

#5 Many notable persons, such as Henry Kissinger and Alexander Haig, had CABG more than ten years ago and seem to be doing well. How do you explain this, and can similar or better results be obtained from Chelation Therapy?

One prominent cardiologist said "the best that can be said for most CABG procedures is that it is irrelevant to the natural course of the disease."

Henry Kissinger, according to a report by Graboys, was admitted to Massachusetts General Hospital because of pain in his right shoulder. The pain was diagnosed as bursitis. Because they wanted to do a thorough job, a cardiac consultation was made, and it was decided that he should have angiography (catheterization) done to study his coronary arteries. Once a blockage is found with angiography, it is difficult to resist the pressure to do surgery to correct it. This was indeed the case for Dr. Kissinger, and surgery was performed. Unfortunately, Dr. Kissinger still had his right shoulder pain when he checked out of the hospital.

Graboys stated in a workshop at the November 1991 meeting of the American College of Advancement of Medicine that, in his experience, many people who claim that they are doing well after CABG surgery feel like they are doing well because they are told they were going to die if they didn't have the surgery, and thus they are happy to be alive. In an average case, CABG surgery needs to be repeated after seven to ten years. These gentlemen may have done very well with their CABG, but they may also need a repeat procedure one of these days. In general, the second operation is riskier than the first. Not knowing the details of their cases, I cannot be sure, but it is possible that they might have done at least as well with Chelation Therapy.

#6 How do the complications following CABG compare with those following Chelation Therapy?

The biggest complication with CABG is a 5-percent risk of death on the table. Some centers will claim a lower mortality figure. The reason might be that they do not operate on people who have severe coronary artery disease with complications. If you operate on a high percentage of relatively well people, you don't expect to have many complications.

One of the most disturbing side effects of CABG is a complaint that many patients have that they don't function as well mentally and their memory is worse after having the surgery and being on the heart-lung machine. Some patients have continuing chest pain, despite having the surgery. This may be due to continuing Coronary Artery Disease or to the scar tissue that results from the surgery.

In contrast, Chelation Therapy has very few side effects, and the ones that occur are of minimal significance. Sometimes there is a temporary lowering of the blood sugar or the blood calcium level that can cause weakness or muscle spasm. This is readily corrected by dietary measures or by giving a brief nutritional injection. There is a slight risk of kidney problems with Chelation Therapy, if the doctor administering the treatment does not carefully follow the standard protocol. The risk results from too much of the EDTA being given too fast and the kidneys become overloaded with toxic metals. This can be tested for, monitored, and corrected in virtually every case. Actually, kidney function improves with Chelation Therapy in most cases, because the circulation to the kidneys is improved.

Several years ago, the American College of Advancement in Medicine estimated that at least 500,000 patients have received Chelation Therapy treatments using the guidelines published in their protocol. This amounts to ten million treatments without a single fatality attributable to EDTA. This undoubtedly makes EDTA Chelation Therapy one of the safest treatment methods in modern medicine.

#7 What do surgeons say to convince patients to submit to bypass surgery?

Frequently surgeons are trained to take aggressive measures to try to correct problems. If they find blockages in the coronary arteries, then they are anxious to open those blockages. Too often cardiovascular surgeons do not fully explain the good survival rates and low risks associated with continuing on medical therapy rather than undergoing surgery. Instead, they sometimes make generalizations such as "you're probably going to die if you don't have bypass." It is hard to have the fortitude to tell a surgeon that you want to wait and make up your mind slowly if he has told you that you may die without the surgery. Very rarely is there such an emergency that bypass needs to be done on an urgent basis. I believe that any patient who has vascular disease due to hardening of the arteries should be informed about Chelation Therapy as an option for treatment. To withhold chelation as an option is not to get true informed consent.

#8 Numerous other alternatives to Coronary Artery Bypass Graft Surgery have been used experimentally in recent years, such as laser surgery, rotoectomy, and a combination of diet, yoga, and exercise. How do the results of these compare with Chelation Therapy?

Laser surgery and rotoectomy are experimental procedures, although the laser procedure has been approved for certain selected cases just recently. So far, there is no evidence that these procedures are any more beneficial than balloon angioplasty or CABG.

Dean Ornish in California has published results that have shown that with a very strict diet and exercise program, you can improve coronary circulation. I would certainly recommend that people try this approach if they are motivated to do it. However, it is important to recognize that this is a very strict regimen that has to be maintained for the rest of the patient's life. Most people simply do not have the discipline to accomplish these results.

Although Chelation Therapy is also considered "experimental" by conventional medicine, there is a 1989 *Textbook on EDTA Chelation Therapy,* edited by Elmer Cranton, M.D., that gives evidence that EDTA therapy has significantly better results than dietary measures alone. The meta-analysis that Dr. Stahl and I conducted offers very strong evidence that EDTA is related to improvement in vascular disease. However, a detailed study comparing EDTA to lifestyle changes has not been done. My feeling is that the best approach is to combine the best that the patient can do in choosing a healthy diet and regular exercise with the added benefit of Chelation Therapy.

#9 If chelation is so good, why isn't everyone using it?

The simple answer is that most doctors do not believe that chelation works. They have gained that opinion from the medical editorials that have been written against chelation and by the positions of such groups as the AMA and the American Heart Association. Most doctors who read the comprehensive literature on chelation and talk to patients and physicians who are involved in receiving and giving the therapy are convinced that it is an option that should be utilized much more in the treatment of cardiovascular disease. For a detailed answer to this question, I refer you to Dr. James Carter's excellent book *Racketeering in Medicine.*

#10 There is a general public ignorance about Chelation Therapy as a treatment for CABG. Can you explain this?

Chelation Therapy is done by a small minority of physicians in the United States. Even though they are very busy in their practices, they have attempted to do office-based research and a number of good studies have been done. Unfortunately these studies have not been accepted in the major medical journals that most doctors read. The standard therapy for vascular disease is surgery and drugs. This is what has been publicized in the scientific journals as well as the lay press. Such organizations as the American Heart Association have scorned Chelation Therapy, without carefully looking at the evidence. Editorials have been written in such journals as the *Journal of the American Medical Association (JAMA)* against Chelation Therapy without even a cursory examination of the hundreds of articles that have been written in the scientific journals that support Chelation Therapy. There have been a number of excellent books written about Chelation Therapy, however. A large number of patients who have read these books or heard about the results from other patients and who have taken the therapy themselves have benefitted from it.

#11 Why did the FDA raid the office of Dr. Jonathan Wright? Are you afraid of a similar raid?

In the spring of 1992, the FDA made a frightening raid, with guns drawn, on Dr. Jonathan Wright's office. They confiscated some B vitamins that did not contain preservatives and some allergy testing equipment. They terrorized the patients and the staff. There have been numerous newspaper editorials and radio shows that strongly condemn this action by the FDA. Thousands and thousands of letters were written to Congressional representatives about this. I would hope that the FDA would not continue to use such Gestapo tactics. Even though I do not expect a raid to take place in our office, I do not blame my staff for being apprehensive. Only by concerted efforts from all of our friends and patients who strongly protest such actions and try to influence Congress to pass laws forbidding them, can we be safe from such arbitrary and police-state-type raids with little or no justification. Recently, all charges against Dr. Wright were dropped.

#12 How about medical board sanctions?

There have been several state medical boards that have tried to take action against Chelation Therapy, but only a very few have succeeded. Recently, at least seven states have passed laws that forbid the medical board to take actions against doctors who are doing alternative medicine (including Chelation Therapy) as long as there is no demonstrable harm to the patient. In other states, medical boards have been forced to back down on efforts to forbid Chelation Therapy because of legal actions by the doctors involved. In a few states, hearings on Chelation Therapy have convinced the medical board that no action should be taken against it. As a doctor, I am licensed by the medical board in the state in which I practice. I try to keep them informed about the scientific basis of the controversial therapies that I employ in my practice. I believe that this is a reasonable approach and that reasonable people will respond appropriately. But there still are states in which medical boards are acting arbitrarily and capriciously against Chelation Therapy without any evidence that their actions are appropriate.

#13 Why such a detailed "informed consent"?

It is important that each patient realizes that chelation is not a therapy that is considered usual and customary. Whenever such a therapy is given, the patient has a right to know and the physician has the duty to inform the patient of all risks, of the potential benefits and of the alternatives that may be possible to treat whatever condition is present. I explain this to my patients orally, but it helps to have a written consent to which they can refer back in the future. A detailed written consent also helps me to avoid forgetting part of it in my explanation.

#14 What objections do the AMA and other conventional medical organizations have against Chelation Therapy?

Most editorials that have criticized EDTA Chelation Therapy for vascular disease use a combination of three arguments: that there is no proof of its effectiveness, that it is dangerous, and that it is costly.

I have already mentioned a good many articles that have shown the effectiveness of EDTA treatment. It is true that a large double-blind study on EDTA in vascular disease has not been completed. After many hours of work and several years of time, a few key leaders of ACAM (especially Ross Gordon, M.D., in consultation with Emeritus Professor of Georgetown University, Martin Rubin, Ph.D.) worked with the FDA and several funding sources to design and begin such a study. Unfortunately, politics and red tape have coupled to stop the progress of that study. As of this writing, the study is still alive but is inactive.

It should be emphasized that no double-blind study on bypass has been done either. One single-blind, cross-over study by Carter and Olszewer showed dramatic improvement with Chelation Therapy. Previously, I spoke about the Danish cardiovascular surgeons' study that was published in two U.S. medical journals in 1991-92. Besides the fact that most patients in that study continued to smoke, there were many other problems with that study. The study was strongly criticized in an editorial in the *Journal of Advancement in Medicine.* It is interesting to note that the study was done soon after the Danish chelating doctors offered chelation to patients who were on the waiting list for bypass surgery or for amputation, and 82 out of 92 patients who chose to take chelation subsequently canceled their surgery. The meta-analysis at the end of this book discusses 40 articles about the relationship between EDTA therapy and improved cardiovascular function.

For anyone to state that there is no evidence that EDTA Chelation Therapy works is a great distortion of the truth. To say that an expensive rigorous large-scale scientific study has not yet been done is accurate.

Regarding safety, if EDTA is given according to ACAM's protocol, it is safer than aspirin. EDTA is listed on the FDA's GRAS (Generally Regarded As Safe) list. When the FDA was helping set up the study with ACAM's doctors, they recognized so much evidence that EDTA was safe that they stated that further studies were unnecessary. It is true that EDTA might cause kidney damage if it is given in a much greater dose than is currently recommended. In fact, however, EDTA given intravenously usually improves kidney function, according to an article by McDonagh, Cheraskin and Rudolph. Critics sometimes list other potential side effects of chelation, but they almost always fail to point out that they are so infrequent that a doctor doing Chelation Therapy according to the standard protocol all of his professional life would very likely not encounter any of those potential side effects. EDTA is in much of the food we eat and in I.V.s in the hospital in small amounts. It is one of the safest substances available!

Finally, I want to speak about cost. EDTA is so much cheaper than CABG there is no comparison. By getting an intravenous infusion in an office setting, the patient usually pays one-third to one-fourth what he or she would be billed for the same service in a hospital emergency room or outpatient facility. When you consider what you are getting for your money, EDTA is one of the greatest medical bargains available in the world today!

#15 What are the current costs of CABG and Chelation Therapy, including long-range maintenance?

In 1989, a typical CABG operation cost between $30,000 and $40,000 dollars, with additional costs due to subsequent medications that were required and repeat operations in later years, which are often necessary. In 1992 the cost of a CABG in California was $100,000. In 1985, Dr. Harrison found that an average additional expenditure on CABG after the surgery over the next five years was in excess of $32,000. A similar figure of $27,000 was found after angioplasty, which does not include the cost of the frequently required repeat procedures. The angioplasty procedure itself costs around $16,000 (in 1990). This also does not figure in costs that may be related to risk of death, complications from the procedure, and the cost of disability when patients become medically disabled despite their surgical procedures. If you figure in a monetary factor for all these factors, the cost of surgical intervention is probably at least $300,000 over a five- to ten-year follow-up period.

Chelation Therapy costs approximately $80 to $120 per treatment and 30 treatments is a typical course, although patients with more severe problems may require 40 or 50 treatments. Many patients do remain on a maintenance schedule, usually about one treatment a month. There are also costs for monitoring laboratory work, but medications are usually significantly reduced, if not eliminated, after the use of Chelation Therapy. My estimation of total costs over a similar period of time, figuring in risk of disability and so forth, is that Chelation costs one-third to one-sixth as much as CABG.

It must be emphasized that these are estimates. Recently the

Great Lakes Association of Clinical Medicine (GLACM), under the direction of James Carter, M.D., of Tulane University Medical School, has proposed conducting a study comparing the costs of Chelation Therapy with bypass surgery in four countries: the United States, the Netherlands, Denmark, and New Zealand. When this study is completed there will be a definitive answer to the question of cost-effectiveness. GLACM has also released a white paper, "The Cost Effectiveness of Alternative Medicine in the Workplace," which discusses cost issues with Chelation Therapy in more detail. A copy can be obtained from the Executive Director of the Great Lakes Association of Clinical Medicine at 1407-B North Wells Street in Chicago, Illinois 60610.

In 1993, a 62-year-old man came to me for Chelation Therapy. During the previous three years he had spent an average of 130 days per year in the Coronary Care Unit. He had had five heart attacks. He underwent 32 heart catheterizations, one bypass, and seven separate balloon procedures. He required four shots of a powerful narcotic, meperidine (Demerol) to marginally control his pain. After only seven chelation treatments, he was totally off Demerol, he went bowling for the first time in years, and he went on a two-mile hike. His insurance had paid close to one million dollars with lousy results. After investing about $5,000 of his own money on chelation treatments, since his insurance company refused to pay for the therapy, he was finally on the road to recovery.

#16 Why are supplemental vitamins, minerals, and herbs used in conjunction with Chelation Therapy?

Chelation Therapy removes some good minerals from the body as well as the toxic ones. These have to be replaced with oral supplements and by adding some minerals to the I.V. solution itself. Doctors who practice Chelation Therapy are interested in providing the most effective treatments that they can for their patients. Most of these physicians are experts in the nutritional field, and they add vitamins and herbs that have been shown to have additional positive effects on the circulatory system. These nutritional programs are usually individualized, and will vary a great deal from patient to patient.

#17 How is diet used to supplement Chelation Therapy?

The diet is very important in the total program which involves Chelation Therapy. Fats of all kinds must be reduced, but particularly saturated fats which are found in dairy products and meats. Any fat that is cooked or processed is found to be hazardous, even polyunsaturated fats. Refined carbohydrates are also important to avoid, particularly sugar. Depending on the situation, physicians may require further carbohydrate restriction in order to reduce the fats in the blood of the patient. It is also important to avoid too much salt and food additives. The fresher the fruits and vegetables the better.

#18 Why are Chelation Therapy treatments given once or twice a week? Why do they take 3 to 4 hours to be completed?

When Chelation Therapy was first given, it was given every day in the hospital. They gave up to three times the current dose and they administered it over fifteen minutes or so. With that treatment protocol, two patients died of kidney damage because their kidneys were overloaded with the EDTA, which was attached to toxic minerals. The ACAM protocol guards against this successfully by reducing the frequency to once or twice a week or three times in selected cases and by carefully adjusting the dose according to kidney function. With full-dose chelation, it is important that the intravenous be given over at least a three-hour period. Half of the EDTA goes through the body in an hour, so that it is easy to see that chelation is safer with the modern protocol.

Interestingly enough, Dr. Edward McDonagh, who used to do Chelation Therapy in hospitals, observed that the concomitant use of exercise in out-patients getting Chelation Therapy is very beneficial. Patients who received the therapy in an office setting and used an exercise program did much better than those who were treated in the hospital.

#19 What percentage of patients are improved after Chelation Therapy?

Two large studies have been published or are in the process of being published. The first, authored by Drs. Olszewer and Carter, involved 2,500 patients who had heart disease, carotid artery disease, and peripheral vascular disease. Eighty-five to 90 percent of those patients showed a measurable improvement in their disease. The Cypher Study, authored by Drs. Phil Hoekstra, Al Scarchilli, Paul Parente, and others, used thermography to measure small vessel circulation in the legs, arms, and carotid arteries before and after chelation. The Cypher study showed that between 80 and 85 percent of patients had measurable improvements in their circulation. Even some patients who did not demonstrate significant improvement had a reduction in spasm, and they noticed improvement in their functional status. Details of both of these studies can be found in the meta-analyses at the end of this book.

#20 Why do the remaining 10 to 15 percent not receive similar benefits?

We do not know all the answers for every patient. However, there are some patients that do better with the addition of certain nutrient therapies, such as vitamins and herbs. There are some patients who do not respond no matter what you do, and this is true of just about every therapy known to medicine.

#21 Does Chelation Therapy work differently for people of varying age groups?

Chelation Therapy has been beneficial in many patients who are in their 90s as well as in children. In fact, Chelation is used in children who have lead toxicity to remove the lead from their bodies. The chance of benefit in someone greater than 85 years of age might be slightly less than in those patients who are younger, but there is still an excellent chance of good improvement in elderly patients.

#22 Is Chelation Therapy supplemented by additional drip therapy?

Sometimes a patient will get behind in the normal minerals when undergoing Chelation Therapy. Most commonly, this occurs when the patient is depleted of minerals prior to entering therapy (i.e. from diuretics or water pills) or when he or she does not take the oral supplements prescribed by the doctor as directed. The doctor may elect to boost them with a mineral I.V. Other times, doctors will use different I.V.s from time to time to help with other related problems such as hyperlipidemia or unrelated problems such as arthritis. These may be added to the chelation solution or they may be given separately.

#23 Are mineral I.V. supplements necessary for all chelation patients?

Many physicians who use Chelation Therapy do not give mineral I.V.s. Others feel this can be an important adjunct. In our office, we provide the mineral I.V.s in selected patients, mainly to replace minerals that may have been washed out excessively by EDTA. Patients may have been depleted of trace minerals before they began the therapy. This can usually be detected by the various mineral analyses that are done during the testing process, especially the urinary excretion of minerals. When mineral I.V.s are indicated, a standard solution may be given, or additional minerals may be added, depending on the patients laboratory data. When needed, mineral I.V.s are often given every five treatments, but there are a few people who require them even more often than that.

Many patients do well with a mineral I.V. periodically throughout their course of treatments. If patients feel fatigued with their treatments, they should definitely bring that to their physicians' attention in case a mineral I.V. would be indicated.

#24 Why are supplemental I.V.s necessary when supplements are also taken orally?

There is a great deal of variability as far as the efficiency of digestion and absorption. Some people will readily absorb oral supplementation and others do so poorly. Again, the culprit may be oral diuretics, which can lower the body's supply of potassium and magnesium and sometimes trace minerals as well.

#25 What testing is done to measure the effectiveness of Chelation Therapy?

First, there has to be some objective measure of the vascular status of the patient before and after the basic course of treatments. Many times doppler or related testing is used to measure circulation to the carotid arteries or to the legs. Sometimes thermography is used, which measures small vessel circulation as opposed to the larger vessel circulation measured by the doppler. An ultrasound might be done to measure the anatomy of the vessel and, if there is plaque, to determine the percent of narrowing. Sometimes ulcerative plaques can be detected in the carotid arteries, which are more hazardous and usually respond very well to Chelation Therapy.

For the heart, cardiac stress testing is often used, as well as a resting or exercise echocardiogram, cardiac ultrasound, Adenosine or Thallium Stress Tests or other newer tests. In most cases, using non-invasive vascular tests, significant improvements can be demonstrated before and after treatment.

At our clinic, we also like to look at other testing to measure the mechanism of action as we proceed through the treatment. At least every ten I.V.s we measure the tendency of the blood to clot with clotting studies such as the PT, the PTT and Platelet Aggregation. We measure calcium levels before and after treatment to make sure there is a drop in calcium, which shows us the EDTA is working. We like to measure changes in blood fats, both the good cholesterol (HDL), the bad cholesterol (LDL), and the more accurate sub-fractions such as Apo A-1, Apo B, and Lp(a). We expect to see elevated ferritin levels (too much iron) drop, and an increased clotting tendency (as measured by high fibrinogen levels) improve. If most of these measures are improving as we go, then we are confident that the treatments are working as they are supposed to work.

#26 Why aren't treadmill tests and catheterizations done to measure progress?

Sometimes treadmill tests are done, but the more elaborate treadmill tests, using radioactive materials, are usually not required. Catheterizations are rarely done before and after therapy because they are not the best measure of improvement, since they are only two-dimensional and, too frequently, doctors who read the same catheterization have different interpretations. The tests also carry a certain measure of risk of death as well as complications and they are very expensive. Most patients don't want to have these any more than are necessary. Catheterizations look at anatomy while better tests for our purposes are ones that look at function. For example, it takes an improvement of only one-sixth or 15 percent in the diameter of a vessel to double the blood flow through that vessel. A functional test that measures blood flow such as a doppler test may be more important to a patient than an anatomical test.

#27 But wouldn't these tests, effectively passed, and showing improvement in blood flow, silence critics of Chelation Therapy?

It is true that the "gold standard" of coronary artery disease is a catheterization or angiogram. I think it is far too often that standard medicine pays more attention to anatomy than function. People with significant blockages in several coronary arteries may be able to function perfectly well without symptoms or without fear of premature death. Because EDTA's major effect on the plaque is to make it softer and the walls of the arteries more flexible, there may not be significant changes on angiograms. However, there have been cases reported in the literature that do show significant improvement on angiograms and ultrasound testing that do look at anatomy.

#28 Does chelation help small blood vessels more than large ones?

I believe that there is a greater improvement in functional circulation to human tissue than can be demonstrated by angiograms and other large vessel studies. Chelation makes the walls of the vessels softer and more flexible so that more blood can go through. It also acts at the cell membrane level. Thus, I believe that chelation has its greatest effect in the smaller blood vessels. This is harder to measure, but it is also more important as far as getting the maximum blood flow to the target organ which is in greatest need.

#29 Compare the accuracy of the doppler test to coronary artery angiograms.

While doppler tests show function and coronary artery angiograms are more likely to show anatomy, both tests are relatively accurate, but both are also subject to significant differences when submitted to different interpreters. More recent evidence indicates that the function of the left ventricle of the heart is a far more accurate indicator of prognosis than the number and amount of vessel blockages on the coronary angiogram.

#30 What is the relationship of such drugs as beta blockers to Chelation Therapy? Do such drugs enhance or diminish the results of Chelation?

There is some indication that propranolol (Inderal) blocks the action of the parathyroid glands which are needed to mobilize calcium in soft tissue after the level of calcium drops in the blood stream. Most of the time it is suggested that Inderal and other beta blockers be switched to a cardio-selective beta blocker such as atenolol (Tenormin) that should not have this effect on the parathyroid glands.

#31 What is the attitude of insurance companies generally about Chelation Therapy?

There is movement in two directions by different companies.

More and more insurance companies are agreeing to pay for Chelation Therapy as an alternative to bypass surgery because of the cost and safety to the patient. On the other hand, with the financial crunch that insurance companies are experiencing, they are covering fewer medical procedures all the time. Often, the less broadly accepted procedures are the first ones that they refuse to pay.

Generally speaking, we tell our patients not to expect their insurance companies to pay for the procedure, but there are certainly some companies who do pay for it. Patients may be more likely to have insurance coverage if we find evidence of toxic heavy metals as a cause of a person's vascular disease, but it is not uncommon for such evidence to be rejected by review committees.

The chief executives of at least two major insurance companies have expressed privately that they are strongly in favor of Chelation Therapy but that government regulations have forbidden them to offer coverage for it, particularly in co-insurance policies that are supposed to cover the amount that Medicare does not cover.

What will be covered under any National Health Plan that may be proposed can of course only be speculated. Chelation for vascular disease can be a covered service under Britain's National Health Plan. New Zealand is considering a similar move.

#32 Why haven't physicians using Chelation Therapy insisted on double-blind studies comparing Chelation to CABG and/or treatment of Coronary Artery Disease with drugs?

In the first place, no double-blind studies about CABG have ever been done, and certainly there is no convincing proof that it is more effective than medical therapy. Chelation doctors have insufficient political clout to insist on such a comparison study.

On the other hand, several years ago when the AMA Board of Directors was about to vote to condemn Chelation Therapy, Dr. Garry Gordon of ACAM convinced them that there was no basis for doing that. Instead of condemning Chelation Therapy they called upon the chelation doctors to do large scale double-blind studies. It was assumed that this would be impossible because such a study for a new drug to be approved generally costs about 250 million dollars. Certainly doctors in private practice couldn't raise anywhere near that amount of money. Fortunately, with the AMA making this statement calling for more research, the FDA began working with chelation doctors, headed by Drs. Ross Gordon, James Frackelton, and Marty Rubin. With the support of several foundations, the FDA cooperated with the chelation doctors to set up a double-blind study on chelation that has not been completed.

It is difficult to do a double-blind study on EDTA by itself because the I.V. hurts, whereas a placebo would not hurt. Therefore, it would be easy for patients to determine which of them were given the I.V.s with EDTA and which received placebos. The FDA showed their willingness to cooperate by allowing the study to proceed with magnesium added to both the EDTA and the placebo solutions. In this way, neither treatment hurt significantly. This was an unusual step by the FDA and was greatly appreciated by the chelation physicians. The meta-analysis chapter at the end of this book discusses other single and double-blind studies on EDTA that have been done or are in progress.

#33 Can you give specific examples of efforts made by chelation physicians to have such studies made?

Such studies have been envisioned by chelation doctors since the mid-1970s, but previous efforts to get them funded and approved met with obstacles. Dr. Ross Gordon and the organization he heads, called the American Institute for Medical Preventics, worked with the FDA over a six-year period to get the studies going in three government hospitals. In the fall of 1991, those studies stalled, partly because the Persian Gulf War efforts drew so many resources away from the hospitals. A major pharmaceutical company at the time committed six and one half million dollars to move the studies into the private sector but since then has reneged on their commitment. At this time, alternative funding is being sought.

#34 Is there currently a study comparing Chelation Therapy to CABG at numerous Veterans Hospitals?

The study involving Chelation Therapy will likely be moved into the private sector as I mentioned. This study does not compare Chelation to CABG. The only study that I know of that makes that comparison is the cost-effectiveness study proposed by Dr. Carter.

#35 Surely some preliminary results have been reported. If so, what do they indicate?

The code has not been broken for the FDA-approved study. However, in the world literature, there have been many studies reported about EDTA Chelation Therapy, and a good number of them have occurred in the United States. They are summarized in the appendices.

With one exception (the study by vascular surgeons in Denmark), all of the multi-patient studies that have been reported have shown the effectiveness of EDTA Chelation Therapy for vascular disease.

Most of them show a measurable improvement of 80 to 90 percent of the patients treated. There was a double-blind study by Drs. Olszewer and Carter reported in the *National Medical Association Journal.* It was a small study of ten patients, but all of the five patients who were treated with EDTA improved, and none of the placebo patients improved. When the code was broken, the untreated patients were subsequently treated with EDTA. They then improved as well.

There have been a number of studies by Drs. McDonagh, Rudolph, and Cheraskin and others that have shown various positive effects of EDTA, including effects on the cholesterol, on pulmonary function, on a feeling of well-being, on clotting mechanisms, and on various non-invasive testing techniques.

The McDonagh studies have been published in a monograph entitled "A Collection of Published Papers Showing the Efficacy of EDTA Chelation Therapy," available from the McDonagh Medical Center, Inc., at 2800A Kendellwood Parkway, Gladstone, Missouri 64119. They showed a significant drop in the cholesterol and a rise in the HDL (or good cholesterol) in treated patients. Kidney function, vascular blood flow, pulmonary function, and bone density were shown to improve. Even patients with psychiatric symptoms tended to get better with treatment, although the cause of this improvement is not known.

#36 Are there other studies, not considered anecdotal, that can be used to make the case for Chelation Therapy over CABG?

All of the studies that I have mentioned are scientific studies that have statistical significance. The Carter and Olszewer study of 2,800 patients showing an 85-percent improvement is a very significant study, as is the Cypher Study, which contained 19,000 patients and had similar results. Using the statistical technique of meta-analysis, we put all of these studies together and an even higher degree of statistical significance resulted.

#37 About what percentage of your patients have come to you as a result of failed CABG?

I would estimate that 15 to 20 percent of my patients would fit into this category. It is exciting to note that even if the patient has had several surgical procedures and a surgeon has told him/her that nothing more can be done surgically, Chelation Therapy can often be very beneficial.

#38 Can you describe a typical case?

A typical case would be a man in his 60s who has developed chest pain and has a positive exercise EKG. Because he was fortunate enough to have gone to a doctor who fully described the potential dangers and potential benefits of the surgical approach, he is very apprehensive that the surgical approach may not be completely successful.

The patient has read something about Chelation Therapy and is interested, although some of his relatives object because of not following the standard line of medicine. The patient has brought test results that had been done previously. Further testing is done to update this material. The risks and benefits of Chelation Therapy are explained to the patient and he starts treatment with a sense of hopefulness but also with some sense of skepticism.

The patient is encouraged by the number of reports that he hears from his fellow patients as he is getting his I.V.s, because so many of them are very willing to talk about the improvements that they have experienced.

Some patients may start to feel better fairly quickly after beginning treatments, but, more likely, our patient notices a significant change after 10 or 15 treatments.

At that point, the nitroglycerine that he was required to take before becomes less and less necessary. His blood pressure is easily controlled and his exercise ability increases significantly. By the end of a typical course of 30 treatments, he is taking a minimum amount of medication and has returned to a more vigorous lifestyle, which may mean resuming work full time.

There may be changes noticed that he didn't expect, such as being able to see a little more clearly, or being able to hear a little more acutely. We see unexpected changes very frequently. The patient is then eager to maintain his nutritional supplements and to schedule monthly booster treatments to insure that his health improvements continue.

#39 What have been the results—both long-range and short-range—of this typical patient?

Short-range, the cholesterol dropped 100 points, the HDL rose 10-15 points, the clotting studies showed a significantly decreased tendency to clot, the calcium blood levels dropped temporarily. The patient noticed a change in the texture of his skin. It is softer and healthier. In the long range, he has a much more vigorous life style with a significant improvement in the way he feels. He is less prone to heart attacks and strokes, and generally enjoys life to a much fuller extent.

#40 What part does mental attitude play with Chelation Therapy?

Certainly, mental attitude is a positive way that people can help contribute to their improvement and reduce stress. A positive attitude and peace of mind all add to the general well-being of a patient. Although the hard-driving Type A people cannot change their basic personalities, they can make a few adjustments that will reduce the stress impact. Thus they function better and their blood will clot less easily.

I believe that any treatment is likely to be more successful if the patient agrees with the treatment and submits to it enthusiastically. Norman Cousins, in *Anatomy of an Illness,* demonstrated that a positive mental attitude can have a tremendous benefit on various illnesses. Therefore, I think it is very important to do everything possible to foster such an attitude in our patients. On the other hand, the effects of EDTA and magnesium in the chelation solution have a benefit that goes well beyond any that could be expected from just a positive mental attitude.

#41 What kind of water should I drink? Is distilled water important?

The majority of the body's makeup is water. It is very

important that we have a good source of high-quality water and that we drink plenty of it to flush the body and provide the new fluids that we need. Unfortunately, some water is toxic. Pesticides, heavy metals, and other toxic substances are routinely found in most water sources. Chlorine has some possible detrimental effects and certainly nobody should drink softened water on a regular basis due to the high sodium content.

Therefore, the best recommendation of most physicians who give Chelation Therapy is that a patient drinks six to eight glasses of distilled water per day. The extra water enables the blood to flow more freely and also makes the urine more dilute, which is easier on the kidneys, especially if heavy metals are being removed by EDTA. Since grocery store sources of distilled water are contained in plastic jugs which can leach additional toxic substances, it is probably best to use your own water purification system at home. One must remember that if one is drinking distilled water on a regular basis, it is mandatory that he or she replaces trace minerals through a multivitamin preparation. Some people feel that their well water is of high quality, but they should not rely on taste alone. Those who are not using a water purification system should have their water tested to see how safe it is. In our area of the country, the water tends to be very hard. It is very high in calcium and iron. Too much of these minerals can be toxic to the body and increase the development of vascular disease.

#42 Why is distilled water recommended over spring water or purified water like that available in supermarkets?

There have been some questions about the degree of purification in so-called "purified" water. It is very difficult to verify purity in water that you get from the grocery store, although generally speaking, I think that purified water from the grocery store is better than tap water.

The best way is to use a reverse osmosis or comparable purification system in your own home. That way you are confident that the job is done well and you are getting the best water possible.

#43 If I am traveling while undergoing chelation treatments, can I continue treatments elsewhere?

Physicians who belong to ACAM agree to abide by the same basic protocol, with individual variations. The doctors who are listed in the directory as diplomates have undergone additional testing and certification procedures to assure that they are experts in the field. I would be comfortable referring my patients to most members of ACAM, especially if I know them personally or if they have achieved diplomate status. We are always happy to share our records with colleagues so that patients can get the best medical care available wherever they are.

#44 How can I find a reputable chelation doctor who will continue my treatments?

ACAM has a national directory of doctors who perform Chelation Therapy to a specified standard. ACAM's address is 23121 Verdugo Drive, Laguna Hills, CA 92653 (toll-free at 800-532-3688). I think you can rely on their recommendation quite well, although I am also happy to give my personal recommendation to those who might inquire through our office.

#45 How can I be sure that the treatments I am getting in another location are the same as those I receive from you?

I am always happy to share my prescribed formula with another physician. In most cases, the physician is able to duplicate that formula if he is a member of ACAM or the Great Lakes Association of Clinical Medicine (toll-free at 800-286-6013). However, each doctor has to use his own clinical judgement and he may be more comfortable with a very slight variation on what I use for one reason or another. You need to establish a rapport with the doctor involved and make the decision together.

#46 Can you cite patients who have completed an initial Chelation Therapy (the full cycle) and who are willing to testify to the effectiveness of their treatment?

I provide my patients with a list of patients who are willing to talk to others who are interested in Chelation Therapy. It is my hope that each doctor who provides this book as a reference for patients include his/her own list of patients who are willing to discuss their chelation treatments. Ask your doctor for such a list.

#47 What goes on at the meetings of the American College for Advancement in Medicine (ACAM), and the Great Lakes Association for Clinical Medicine (GLACM)?

These two organizations both conduct scientific meetings of extremely high quality. Some of the more prominent researchers in the world have presented their findings at the meetings of both organizations. Workshops are held by doctors who have a great deal of practical experience in clinical medicine. There is a lot of give and take with doctors searching for suggestions on how they can treat their patients more effectively. Nutritional supplement companies have booths at the meetings and may contribute speakers to discuss what is new in research in the nutritional field. When I come back from a three-or four-day meeting held by one of these organizations, I usually have a list of 20 or more procedures I want to do differently in our office. New therapies, new protocols, and reminders of old therapies that I haven't used lately are some of what we learn at these meetings. All of these can add to my effectiveness as a treating physician. I find them extremely valuable in finding innovative ways to help my patients more effectively.

#48 If you yourself suffered chest pains with a related diagnosis of atherosclerosis, would you take the same treatments you recommend to others?

As a matter of fact, that has already happened. Almost three years ago, I started running with my daughter who was trying to get ready to run cross-country in high school. I started getting chest pains after running two or three blocks. Previously I had received a few Chelation Therapy treatments, but none on a regular basis. I had exercised before, but I hadn't been running for some time.

I had a positive exercise stress test and saw a cardiologist. The recommendation was that I get angiography and be evaluated as to whether bypass surgery would be needed. I took a standard course of Chelation Therapy and gradually increased my exercise tolerance. One year later, I was able to run 18 miles without stopping and without chest pains!

This story is very typical of doctors who practice Chelation Therapy. The vast majority of them take the treatments themselves and offer it to their families and loved ones.

#49 What can a convinced layman do to help open the eyes of those who have been blind to the beneficial effects of Chelation Therapy?

One of the best actions that could be taken would be to convince a legislator to introduce legislation protecting chelation doctors from actions by State Medical Boards, provided there is no demonstrable harm to the patient. This law has been passed by a number of states and is being considered by several others. What it does is ensure that the physician can practice advanced medicine without fear of being harassed and—especially—without the threat of losing his license. In every state where this legislation has been passed, the action was made possible by patients and lay people rather than primary activity by physicians themselves.

Another action might be to spread the word as widely as possible, giving books like this one and other books that have been written about Chelation Therapy to physicians and friends all over the country. The most popular books include several by Dr. Morton Walker, including *Chelation Therapy*, written with John Trowbridge, M.D.; *The Chelation Answer* written with Dr. Garry Gordon; and his latest, *The Chelation Way*. *Bypassing Bypass,* by Dr. Elmer Cranton and Arline Brecher, and Arline's 1992 best-seller, *Forty-Something Forever* have been very popular. This will help people understand how effective the therapy really is.

It would also be helpful to write people associated with newspapers, radio, and T.V. to encourage them to do articles or to interview people who have had Chelation Therapy or doctors who are giving it. Once again, media people will respond to inquiries from the public better than from any contacts from physicians.

You can ask your insurance companies to cover Chelation Therapy and tell them why. It is especially true that insurance companies that insure larger companies will cover anything that negotiations ask them to cover. Most of the time, nobody asks them what specific procedures they want covered. Self-insured groups can often determine what is and what is not covered for them. If insurance companies see that Chelation Therapy might save them some of the ten billion dollars that they spend on bypass surgery each year, they may get interested in a hurry.

#50 What are the most common side effects, if any, of Chelation Therapy?

If the patient were *not* treated with the ACAM protocol, and he received too high a dose more frequently than is safe, he could potentially get some kidney damage. This has not been reported for *any* patient in which the standard protocol was followed. It is still very important that the doctor is well-trained and careful. Sometimes the patient might feel a little tired after the therapy or have a headache that lasts for a short period of time. There may be a little discomfort at the site of the I.V. The blood pressure might dip a little low during the therapy.

If a patient is getting behind in his minerals he might have some cramping or a minor disturbance of heart rhythm. None of these are serious side effects and they can usually be corrected easily with minor adjustments to the therapy.

#51 What are the aftereffects of Chelation?

The biggest aftereffect of chelation is that patients are healthier overall, and they feel better.

#52 What causes the delayed improvement that you sometimes see after a patient has completed a course of Chelation Therapy?

That question has been debated extensively among chelating physicians. For some reason, the body continues to heal itself for at least three months after a basic course of Chelation Therapy has concluded. One explanation might be that trace minerals are replenished gradually during that time period, but that is only a factor in certain patients. Another explanation is that EDTA is basically treating an antioxidant deficiency, not hyperlipidemia. Even elevated LDL cholesterol is harmless unless it is oxidized. We need lots of broad spectrum antioxidants in our system, which we get from vitamin E, beta-carotene, vitamin C, and selenium. EDTA removes the pro-oxidants, or many of the substances that stimulate oxidation in the body. Rust is caused by a similar process of oxidation. In effect, EDTA creates a "rust-proofing" for the body. Once this rust-proofing is applied, the body can continue to heal itself. For this reason, some physicians do not do repeat cardiovascular testing until several months after the basic course of treatment is concluded. However, others will repeat the tests sooner because they want to get a better idea of how many treatments may be needed for a particular patient.

#53 What do you think of oral chelation? Is it as effective as I.V. Chelation Therapy?

There are two types of oral chelation. Sometimes they are combined. The first uses high-dose vitamins and minerals that serve as antioxidants and weak chelators.

The second is the use of oral EDTA. About 5 percent of EDTA is absorbed by mouth. Theoretically, if you took four to six pills of a high-quality oral EDTA you may absorb enough to be equivalent to one treatment a month. However, this is spread over such a long period of time that I doubt that the effect would be as good as an intravenous treatment. The rapid rise and fall of EDTA in the bloodstream may be an important part of the mechanism of action. This can only occur with intravenous use. Oral treatment certainly would not suffice for a basic course of treatment. There is also a possibility that oral EDTA that is not absorbed would hold important minerals in the gut and prevent them from passing into the blood.

There is no scientific proof that oral EDTA or using high-dose vitamin and mineral preparations can do anything to reverse atherosclerosis. I think that the nutrient therapies are good to slow down the disease process and help prevent damage from reoccurring.

#54 Can oral chelation be used as maintenance?

It could be tried. Once again, there is no scientific data to support its use.

#55 Can oral chelation be used between regular weekly chelation treatments?

Yes, it can. It might be beneficial, especially the antioxidant sources mentioned in question #52 and such important minerals as calcium, magnesium, selenium, manganese and chromium. We use the nutrient form of oral chelation routinely as part of our nutritional supplements. We do not use oral EDTA during the treatment time.

#56 Have you ever given up on a coronary artery patient and recommended that he or she submit to CABG surgery?

Yes, I have on rare occasions, when the patient continues to have severe symptoms or disability due to heart function, despite a good treatment program with EDTA and nutritional substances with appropriate lifestyle changes. In the cases that I remember, the patients generally return to me afterwards to get Chelation Therapy following CABG surgery. These patients usually do well.

#57 Describe a worst-case scenario and how you would treat it.

A worst-case scenario might be a patient who is not a surgical candidate, is very weak from depletion of minerals, and has severe coronary artery disease with congestive heart failure.

I would treat this patient with the support of a cardiologist. I would probably alternate mineral I.V.s with EDTA Chelation Therapy and monitor his kidney function very carefully. I would avoid sodium in the I.V.s as much as possible and perhaps use a low-dose diuretic right after the I.V. to get rid of any sodium that was given. Large doses of nutrient therapies, such as vitamins A, E, and C and selenium with co-enzyme Q-10 would be very important. The patient's magnesium/calcium balance would have to be assessed very carefully and other adjustments in the therapy might be needed as well. The patient would be placed on a careful diet, and attempts to minimize stress would be made. It would be a very difficult case, but there would be a reasonable chance of success.

#58 Some people recommend a low-carbohydrate diet and others recommend a high-carbohydrate diet, but with a reduction in refined sugars. How do I know which one works best and which one I should use?

Chelating physicians generally agree that the diet should be low in processed and cooked fats, white sugar, and white flour.

Additives, preservatives, and salt should be avoided. Stimulants such as caffeine should not be used. Alcohol should also not be used, especially near the time of chelation.

The standard diet is similar to the high-carbohydrate diet that is recommended by most physicians to treat diabetes nowadays. However, many physicians who take a holistic approach to vascular disease have adopted a concept that was first proposed by Dr. Robert Atkins in his book *Dr. Atkins' Diet Revolution*, which was popular in the 1970s. (By the way, that book has recently been updated and is probably available in your bookstores.) The low-carbohydrate diet restricts high-fiber carbohydrates such as milk products and certain fruits, beans, and grains, even if they are whole grain products. Dr. Atkins contends that lower carbohydrate intake will reduce insulin production. Increased production of insulin has been shown to be atherogenic, or to be a direct cause of hardening of the arteries. Insulin also acts indirectly by stimulating the liver to produce more carbohydrates.

When someone is consistently on a lower carbohydrate intake, they first get their energy from glycogen stores and then they switch to mobilized fat for energy. In this way, the diet can help people lose weight with a constant flow of energy rather than the ups and downs which you see with a higher carbohydrate intake. Dr. Atkins cautions patients that if they go on and off the diet, they may do worse then being off the diet altogether. The reason for that is they cannot get energy from either glycogen stores or from fat and as a result they feel tired. Some people who feel tired on the low carbohydrate diet actually need to increase their fat intake slightly.

Dramatic reductions in cholesterol and triglycerides and a rise in the HDL (good cholesterol) are often seen within the first month on a low-carbohydrate diet.

Whether a high-complex-carbohydrate diet or a low-carbohydrate diet is recommended is an individual decision that should be made by the physician based on the biochemical problem of the patient. Both of them can be helpful, depending upon the circumstances.

#59 After I start EDTA treatments, when can I increase my activity?

Often the treating doctor will do a stress EKG prior to starting the treatment if the heart is involved. I think it is important for patients to exercise during their chelation treatments. They need to start with a level of aerobic exercise they can do easily and regularly and then gradually build up. After the first week or two of therapy, some people will notice improvements in their ability to exercise. For others it may take longer, but always there should be an effort to gradually increase exercise, while at the same time not pushing yourself to the point of exhaustion or significant chest pain. Your doctor should give you guidance on a safe and effective exercise program.

#60 Should my medicines be reduced when taking Chelation Therapy?

Most patients can have their medications reduced and sometimes eliminated with Chelation Therapy, but those changes should always be done in consultation with your physician. We make changes gradually so that there is no sudden impact to the body. Some patients would prefer to allow their cardiologist to make the medication changes as he or she notes improvement.

#61 Can I get off all my medications?

Some people are capable of functioning very well without any medications after receiving Chelation Therapy and others will require a few continuing medicines. Usually the total amount of medications is reduced, and the patient functions much better.

#62 If my I.V. hurts at the place where the needle is in my arm, what can be done?

Several measures can be taken to help with discomfort from the I.V. itself. The rate of infusion can be slowed down. Heat can be applied to the forearm and the contents of the I.V. solution can be modified by adding some additional local anesthetic or magnesium. Sometimes a patient will react to the preservatives or other ingredients in the treatment bottle. If this is the case, they will improve when the offending agents are omitted from the solution.

#63 I hate to take so many pills! Are they all necessary?

The vitamins and minerals given during Chelation Therapy are given to enhance the results of the therapy, to replace minerals that have been removed but are needed, and for additional therapeutic effects in themselves. These nutrients are given to build you up and not for the purpose of blocking actions of the body like medications do. Thus they are much safer than drugs. Many people do have to take a significant number of vitamins, minerals, and other nutrients but usually when they realize how much benefit they are receiving from this treatment plan, they are happy to continue them.

#64 My family history is bad for heart disease but I seem to be healthy. Should I take chelation as a prevention treatment?

One of the strongest risk factors for heart disease is your family history. If you have a significant family history for heart disease, stroke, or other circulation problems, I think it would be of major benefit to take a series of chelation treatments. The disease is present long before the first symptoms occur and as with any other problem, the earlier you treat it, the better.

According to Dr. Robert Vogel at the University of Maryland, one of the great misconceptions within cardiology is that arterial blockages of less than 50 percent are "normal" or "insignificant."

Forty-six percent of patients with subsequent heart attacks were told they had normal angiograms or stenoses of less than 25 percent, if they had previous coronary angiography. Seven-year survival rates were *the same* in patients with less than 50-percent blockage as for those who had greater than 50-percent stenosis in three or more vessels.

The answer is *not* to do more bypass surgery. I feel it would be much more effective to emphasize preventive measures and to offer chelation to those patients at high risk.

#65 Is caffeine a problem?

There have been conflicting studies about the effects of caffeine on cardiovascular disease, but I strongly believe that caffeine can have an adverse effect. It is a stimulant that can increase the risk of arrhythmias and also raise the levels of glucose in the blood, which results in increased tendency for the blood to clot.

#66 Should I take aspirin along with my chelation treatments?

I usually take people off aspirin and other anticoagulants during the chelation treatment because EDTA itself has a powerful anticoagulant action. However, there are a few patients that I continue on aspirin or other anticoagulants such as Coumadin. I believe it is important to monitor these patients very carefully to make sure they don't receive too much anticoagulant effect. Blood tests are necessary to insure that the combined therapy is safe and effective.

#67 Should I take vitamin E?

There is *strong* evidence that vitamin E taken on a regular basis in the amount of at least 100 units a day is effective in preventing heart disease. In my experience I have found the natural vitamin E to be more effective. Many patients who have symptomatic vascular disease require higher doses. One has to be careful because very high doses of vitamin E can produce toxic effects due to the fact that it is fat-soluble and accumulates in the body. The higher the dose, the more important it is to use a natural source, which seems to be safer. It is not uncommon for me to recommend up to 2,000 units a day of vitamin E when a good anticoagulant effect is needed.

#68 How about fish oils?

Fish oils have been shown to reduce cholesterol and triglycerides when used in large doses. I certainly feel that it is advisable to eat fish two or three times a week, especially if the source is from cold ocean waters. Lower doses of fish oil, such as two or three capsules a day, can be effective in reducing platelet aggregation much in the way aspirin helps to prevent heart attacks or strokes. A drawback might be the accumulation of mercury, PCBs, and other toxins that have been reported in fish.

#69 When is a patient too old to take Chelation Therapy?

Remarkably, I have seen patients in their 90s respond very well to treatments with EDTA chelation. I do not feel that anyone is too old to take Chelation Therapy.

#70 Will it help Alzheimer's disease?

There are no really good treatments for helping Alzheimer's disease. However, Chelation Therapy can improve the circulation to the brain and to whatever extent the problem is due to a circulation deficit, chelation may have significant benefit. It is very difficult to tell in advance which patients are going to be helped, but I have certainly witnessed a good number of cases where dramatic improvements in memory and mental function occur in patients who carry the diagnosis of

Alzheimer's disease. At this time it is difficult to assess how much brain damage has actually occurred in patients with standard tests. Only on autopsies can we be sure about the extent of permanent brain damage present. Therefore, I tell my patients that the chances of success are probably no more than 50 percent, but if it helps, it may help dramatically.

#71 Will chelation help arthritis?

By its antioxidant enhancing effects, EDTA can reduce inflammation and possibly reduce the damaging effects of arthritis. However, the results are not as predictable as they are with vascular disease. I would try oral antioxidants and other nutritional treatments first in the treatment of osteoarthritis, especially if vascular disease is not also present.

#72 Will chelation help Parkinson's disease?

There have been some reports in the literature and I have seen some patients that have improved with Parkinson's disease. Chelation treatment is not nearly as effective with this disease as with vascular disease. I would be hesitant to use chelation as a primary treatment for Parkinson's disease without evidence of coexisting vascular disease.

#73 Can chelation help multiple sclerosis?

EDTA chelation has not been shown to help multiple sclerosis by itself. M.S. is a very difficult disease to treat effectively. It is possible that EDTA could be used along with a number of other modalities in treating M.S. in an experimental treatment design. Once again, the benefit might arise from EDTA's antioxidant effect and its reduction in soft tissue calcium.

#74 Is it a good idea to take lecithin?

Dr. Lester Morrison has done a great deal of research on the beneficial effects of lecithin in controlling cholesterol problems and in controlling cardiovascular disease. I don't always specifically recommend that patients take lecithin regularly, but I have no objections if they do. Many times it can be very helpful to help control cholesterol problems.

#75 What do the different fat fractions mean and how are they important in vascular disease?

First, one must keep in mind that 80 percent of the body's cholesterol is produced in the liver. Only 20 percent comes directly from the diet. It does little good to look at a patient's total cholesterol. To get meaningful information, one needs to know the HDL or High-Density-Lipoprotein, which you want as high as you can get to protect yourself from vascular disease, and the LDL, or Low-Density-Lipoprotein, which, if elevated, is a risk factor for developing hardening of the arteries. It is also important to examine the apo-lipoproteins if there is a problem with the cholesterol. The Apo-A1 fraction has a protective effect and is a major constituent of the HDL. The Apo-B has a detrimental effect and can be toxic in the process of atherogenesis. Finally, the Lp(a) is another sub-fraction of the cholesterol that is toxic. It is important to keep that fraction as low as you can.

There have been a number of articles in the British medical literature recently that have demonstrated that there is no improvement in survival in patients that are on cholesterol-lowering programs. The reasons are not clear. There is a higher incidence of deaths not due to illness—such as suicides and violence. The drugs used may be hazardous. Patients placed on diets may follow them poorly. It is clearly important to look at the whole picture, not just the total cholesterol.

#76 When should I take my packet of vitamins? Should I avoid them on the day of my intravenous treatment? How about within 24 hours after the treatment?

Generally, we provide packets of vitamins that should be taken twice a day to replace the minerals that are lost and to enhance the effects of Chelation Therapy with high-dose vitamins, minerals, and other substances. There is some concern about taking calcium on the day of chelation because EDTA acts to remove calcium. One should keep in mind, however, that half of the EDTA infused into the body passes through the kidneys in an hour. There is certainly controversy about taking vitamins on the day of chelation, but my feeling is that you should probably not take the morning packet on the day of treatment. On the other hand, because so much of the EDTA has already been processed by the body by the time evening comes, I think it is fine to take the evening dose. Then you should resume taking the vitamins on a regular basis the next day.

Some people have digestive problems and do not absorb the vitamins fully. If you have any problem with frequent gas, bloating, diarrhea, or constipation, be sure your doctor is alerted. He/she may want to do some testing to identify the problem and correct it.

#77 Is meditation a useful adjunct in the treatment of vascular disease?

Yes, indeed. Dr. Herbert Benson of Harvard popularized the "relaxation response," which teaches the patient to relax quickly and thoroughly for 20 minutes twice a day and which can be a very useful adjunct in the treatment of hypertension and in the reduction of stress. I strongly advocate that patients use some form of relaxation exercise, and meditation is a good one. I feel that reducing the body's "fight or flight" mechanism creates a likelihood that long-term hardening of the arteries may be lessened and a certain number of catastrophic events, such as heart attacks and strokes, may be avoided. Many experts recommend a progressive relaxation technique for at least twenty minutes a day, but the regularity of the process is more important than the length of time or even the intensity. Also if you use a relaxation technique regularly, it is much easier to put it into effect in times when it is needed acutely.

If you are not sure you can relax effectively, biofeedback training may be extremely helpful. With this technique, you are hooked up to a small machine that measures some automatic body function such as pulse rate, blood pressure, or electrical skin resistance. The machine gives you a signal, or "feedback" when you are improving this function with the relaxation technique you are trying to use. Thus you know when you are doing something right and you can get the benefits rapidly.

#78 Why is iron so important?

Iron increases free radical activity in the body and thus makes it much harder for the body to provide antioxidants sufficient to prevent damage resulting in chronic illness. Thus excessive iron is a risk factor for developing premature aging, heart disease, arthritis, and cancer. It is very important for everyone to know how much iron he has in his body through the ferritin blood test. If it is too high, the amount of iron can be reduced through Chelation Therapy using EDTA or Desferroxamine. Another treatment involves periodically donating blood so that the iron is taken out of the body through the red blood cells.

#79 I understand that Chelation Therapy can affect the entire vascular system. Is there a limit as to what it can do?

It is true that Chelation Therapy seems to affect circulation throughout the body. Every organ in the body depends on circulation to provide nutrients and oxygen that help it function well. Some people believe that EDTA's primary effect is on the smaller vessels of the body, perhaps explaining why the effects we see clinically are sometimes more dramatic than the changes we see on vascular testing that measure the larger vessels. Certainly a number of patients whom I have seen with macular degeneration, which involves the tiny vessels in the back of the eye, have been greatly benefitted by a course of EDTA treatment. The limits of EDTA's beneficial effects in vascular disease are not well known because they are very difficult to study. First, it must be broadly accepted as a vascular treatment and then we may be able to find ways to refine the treatment so that it can be more effective for more difficult conditions.

#80 What is the proper administration time for a bottle of EDTA, according to the protocol of the American Board of Chelation Therapy?

A bottle should be administered over a three- to five-hour period, depending on the patient's kidney function and cardio-vascular status. A few of the published studies have shown benefit with a smaller bottle using a lesser amount of EDTA over a shortened period of time. How much benefit can be gained when using the shorter bottle is not yet known. The Board of ACAM has addressed this controversy and has stated that in individual circumstances there may be reason to use a lesser dose of EDTA. However, when that decision has been made by the physician, the patient should be informed that the standard protocol for use of EDTA, which has withstood the test of time, is not being followed. Some physicians try to use EDTA as a surfactant which results in making all of the fluids in the body more slippery. A different dose of EDTA is used and the ingredients of the I.V. bottle are distinctly different. This is *not* Chelation Therapy as defined by the American College for the Advancement in Medicine.

A recent unpublished study by Grant Born, D.O., and Tammy Geurkink-Born, D.O., showed that you can get significant improvement in blood flow with a short bottle and a 1.5 gram dose instead of the usual 3 grams.

Similar changes in the clotting studies occurred, with both the 1.5 gram and the 3 gram dose, according to the Borns. More work has to be done to give us the final answer in this controversy.

#81 Should patients exercise after Chelation Therapy? If this is important should the exercise be done in an office or during the I.V.?

Dr. Ed McDonagh did Chelation Therapy in the hospital for a number of years before he began using it in his office as an outpatient treatment. He noticed that the results seemed to be quicker and more effective with outpatient therapy. His conclusion was that the sedentary confinement of patients in the hospital had an adverse effect as far as Chelation Therapy went. Patients seemed to do much better if they exercised after the treatment. Some physicians have installed exercise bicycles or other equipment for patients to use very close to their treatments or even during their treatments. In our office, we have found this to be somewhat cumbersome. It may present problems as there can be side effects of low blood sugar or blood pressure during the intravenous treatment. We do recommend, however, that patients get regular exercise of an aerobic nature shortly after the treatment or at least that evening. This can consist of a 20- to 30-minute brisk walk or other suitable aerobic exercise. Other than a general contribution to physical fitness, I do not feel that exercise just prior to an EDTA treatment has been shown to have an additional effect.

#82 Why are there some people who do not respond with improvement after taking Chelation Therapy?

We do not know all the reasons why Chelation Therapy does not seem to work in some patients. However, physicians speculate that these patients may not be making the lifestyle changes in diet and exercise that are required along with the therapy. It is also possible that they do not take enough of their nutritional supplements or they may have some digestive problem whereby they do not absorb their supplements and get the full benefit from them. Other patients may have more severe abnormalities with their clotting mechanisms or other atherogenic factors. More research needs to be done regarding the relatively few people who do not seem to benefit from Chelation

Therapy. As we find the answers, I'm sure that new and better therapies will be developed that will be even more effective than EDTA therapy is now.

#83 How are treatments individualized? How often is this done?

Most patients are begun with the standard protocol advocated by the American College of Advancement in Medicine. That protocol, however, does allow for variances, depending on the patient's condition. For example, if the kidney function is reduced, then a lesser dose of EDTA would be provided. Another problem might be sodium overload, especially in cases of extreme hypertension or congestive heart failure. In such a case every effort would be made to reduce the sodium in the solution. For patients with hypertension or angina, where spasm is a factor, more magnesium may be used in the solution. Heparin is an anti-coagulant that is usually used to prevent phlebitis, but if a patient is using other anti-coagulants, then this may be a hazardous addition. Some patients may not tolerate certain additives to the solution. The most common one not tolerated is B-complex, because of the preservatives contained in the preparation.

In our office, the ingredients in the I.V. are regularly reviewed by the physician. Adjustments are made accordingly. A more extensive review is made when the patient visits with the physician, which occurs at least every ten treatments.

#84 What are the chances of progression of the vascular disease if maintenance therapy is not given?

Dr. Olszewer and his colleagues in Brazil have determined that the best maintenance schedule after a basic course of Chelation Therapy is a treatment every three to four weeks. Most physicians throughout the world now recommend that patients continue on a maintenance schedule with a treatment every month or so. Doctors are more strict with the patients who have had severe illness. Some patients elect to do without maintenance treatments. Many have done well as far as their symptoms go over a period of years. Nevertheless, it is likely that the same process that caused them to develop hardening of the arteries in the first place continues on to a certain extent, even if significant lifestyle changes have been made. It is not a good idea to rely exclusively on symptoms that may or may not be present, because the process of atherosclerosis goes on long before symptoms develop. Sooner or later most patients will probably get worse if they do not take maintenance therapy. The anti-platelet effect of EDTA, which reduces the tendency of the blood to clot, probably lasts no more than 7-11 days because the platelet pool is renewed that often. Since this mechanism is important in the action of EDTA, treatments should be repeated on a maintenance schedule.

#85 Why is sodium used in the I.V. solution?

The most common form of EDTA that is available today is disodium EDTA. This is changed in the bottle to sodium-magnesium EDTA by adding a significant amount of magnesium before the intravenous solution is infused. Theoretically, there could be a danger in getting sodium in an intravenous solution for high-risk patients, especially those with congestive heart failure, although it is certainly done every day in hospitals. Practically speaking, as long as the doctor is careful, there is rarely any problem with using small amounts of sodium in the solution.

#86 Can Chelation Therapy help an aneurysm?

An aneurysm is caused by a weakness in the wall of the blood vessel, resulting in a dilated vessel that can actually leak blood or rupture. This could be a very dangerous situation that may result in hemorrhage. EDTA will not reduce an aneurysm. It may make the walls of the blood vessel healthier, with less of a calcium build-up, but I would not use it as a primary treatment for an aneurysm.

#87 Should milk be consumed while a patient is taking Chelation Therapy?

Generally speaking, milk is an excellent food for baby cows, but it is not an ideal drink for human beings, especially after growth has been completed and especially in its homogenized form. It is better to avoid the fat that is in milk and it is also possible to get too much calcium, especially if it is not balanced with magnesium. There is not a significant amount of magnesium in milk. A further problem is that milk is the most common food allergy. Therefore, we recommend that patients do not drink milk or consume much in the way of dairy products. They can obtain calcium from green vegetables and other food sources. And, of course, we do include calcium with a careful balance of magnesium in the multivitamin preparations that we provide. For patients who have a strong desire to continue consuming milk, the best source is probably yogurt, and some people may get along with a small amount of milk on their cereal, especially if they don't take it everyday. We strongly recommend that patients avoid milk on the days that they chelate. If the patient has a lot of calcium in their system when they are taking Chelation Therapy, then they may be somewhat less likely to remove the minerals that we want to remove and it may be more difficult to lower the serum calcium to get the desired effect from the parathyroid glands.

#88 Is it possible that women who are taking calcium supplements to prevent osteoporosis could be contributing to their heart attacks and strokes?

Yes, this is indeed possible! Hans Selye demonstrated that he could turn rats to stone by giving them enough oral calcium. When calcium is given, it should always be balanced with magnesium, preferably in a one-to-one ratio. In this way, calcium goes to the areas of the body where it is needed, such as in bone, rather then being deposited in soft tissue.

Too much calcium not balanced with magnesium can theoretically result in hardening of the arteries, stiffening of tissue, increased tendency to clot, and even cell death in areas of the body.

#89 Does EDTA have some side benefits that may treat cancer or arthritis?

By the reduction of heavy metals and excessive iron, EDTA is a great help to the body in controlling free-radical reactions. These free radicals increase the likelihood and speed of development of cancer or arthritis if the predisposition is there for these conditions. Therefore, EDTA could have a free-radical benefit for arthritis and cancer. It is important to stress, however, that there is very little in the scientific literature that links EDTA to improvement in these diseases. There is not yet good evidence for the use of EDTA in treating arthritis or cancer, except if the patient also has vascular disease for which treatment might be warranted.

#90 Why does my angina come and go?

Angina is caused by decreased blood flow to the heart muscle from the coronary arteries. Part of this is due to physical blockage of the arteries in question. The rest is due to spasm of these arteries. The blockage does not change much from day to day unless a new clot is formed. Spasms can vary a great deal, depending upon mineral balance across the cell membranes, various hormones, and other substances which can cause the muscles in the vessel wall to contract or relax. Angina is usually triggered by exercise, but there are forms of it that can be caused entirely by stress or even by eating a meal, especially if food allergies are involved.

One reason why angina might come and go is a borderline or low magnesium level in the body, which is not uncommon. One of the first measures we take with angina is to increase the magnesium intake—sometimes we add taurine, which seems to help the magnesium go into the cells more readily and thus be more effective.

#91 Why are recliner chairs used?

A recliner chair is needed in case the patient might have an episode of low blood pressure during the therapy. If this happens, the treatment is to lie back in the reclined position, which raises the feet to a level at least as high as the head. This tends to reverse the drop in blood pressure. Recliner chairs are also comfortable and some people choose to take a nap during the therapy. However, chiropractors warn that sitting for long periods of time in a recliner may not be good for the spine and may irritate pressure points on the body. Thus, we recommend that patients change positions in their chairs several times during their intravenous treatment.

#92 Define "saw-tooth" progress.

People rarely improve their conditions in straight lines. They usually get a little better and then a little worse and then a little better again and a little worse again. This is called a "saw-tooth" pattern and is especially characteristic of improvements seen on a nutritional program, because there are so many factors that play a role in the body's ability to heal.

#93 Does EDTA help varicose veins?

There is no evidence in the scientific literature that I know of that states that EDTA can be successfully used as a therapy for varicose veins, especially when used according to the standard protocol. As stated earlier, there are some physicians who use EDTA in a solution that makes it easier for the blood to flow through the vessels without necessarily having a strong effect on blockage or arteriosclerosis. Theoretically, this "surfactant" therapy may have some benefit in varicose veins.

#94 What determines the cost of the I.V.?

There may be ten or more ingredients in an intravenous EDTA chelation treatment. Vitamins, minerals, and other substances are added in order to make the therapy safe and more effective and to lessen potential side effects. The doctor must also provide at least one nurse to mix the solution and to monitor the patients' progress. Office overhead must be figured in. Small portions of the cost of each I.V. go toward expenses for the doctors and other staff members to attend continuing education meetings, for research activities, and for handouts, seminars, newsletters, and other ways that the doctor uses to provide information about the therapy to others.

#95 Why can't chelation be given at home?

I think it is important that Chelation Therapy be administered very carefully. If someone does not know exactly how to give and how to monitor the treatment, he or she could do some damage. Both the doctor and the doctor's nursing personnel need to be very knowledgeable about the therapy. I do not believe that it can be given at home under normal circumstances. In our office we do not give Chelation Therapy unless a physician is readily available to provide urgent attention in the rare case when it would be needed. It is at least as important for the nurses to be skilled in the administration of Chelation Therapy. Chelation is one of the safest therapies available, if it's given according to the published protocol. If problems occur, they must be dealt with quickly.

#96 How about patient support groups?

One aspect about Chelation Therapy is that you have a built-in support group with the people who are getting the I.V.s at the same time you do. Much discussion, advice, and encouragement takes place during the treatment session. Several efforts have been made to establish a nationwide network for patient support of

Chelation Therapy. I think these are very much needed and I strongly encourage them. At this time the success of such support groups has not been as great in this country as it has in several others, especially in British Columbia and in New Zealand.

#97 What can I do if I cannot afford Chelation Therapy?

If you cannot afford chelation, you need to do the absolute best job you can in maintaining a healthy lifestyle with an excellent diet, regular exercise, and active ways to combat the effects of stress. I would advise you to take a major anti-oxidant formula with vitamins and minerals in it as prescribed by your physician. Perhaps the most important nutrients to take would be vitamin E, beta carotene, and magnesium. A recent study released by Dr. Walt Willett and others at Harvard showed that you can reduce your chances of having a heart attack by about 40 percent if you take Vitamin E daily. Your doctor may also suggest you take a very low dose of aspirin to prevent aggregation of platelets. However, I believe that nothing is more effective than EDTA Chelation Therapy to reduce the dangerous effects of hardening of the arteries and poor circulation to the heart and other organs. Thus, I think it would be wise to try to budget for treatments for the future. If it is going to be a year before you can actually take the treatments, then you must take measures to try to prevent your problem from getting worse while you save money to enable you to take the treatments.

#98 If I can't change to a perfect lifestyle, am I wasting my money in taking chelation?

It is very important to do the best job you possibly can in improving your lifestyle because Chelation Therapy is only part of the total treatment program. However, there have been some benefits shown in patients who received EDTA chelation and who made no positive changes in their lifestyle. Very few people manage to live a *perfect* lifestyle with a rigid diet, total reduction in stress, and daily exercise. Do the best you can and you'll likely reap great benefits, especially if you take chelation for vascular disease.

#99 How do I find heavy metal toxicity and can I use that for a diagnosis?

Probably the best way to detect heavy metal toxicity is to give an EDTA challenge dose and measure the amount of heavy metals that come out into the urine. If there is a high level of metals or a significant increase (usually three-fold) from the baseline level then that is a good indication that there are too many heavy metals built up in the body. Whether this evidence will be enough to convince your insurance company that the chelation treatments should be covered because of heavy metal toxicity is uncertain. Some companies accept the diagnosis if shown in this way, but others have a much stricter criterion that involves finding an elevated blood level of heavy metals. Unfortunately, the latter criterion is very inaccurate because most heavy metals pass quickly out of the blood into the fat, bones, and other storage tissues of the body soon after they are accumulated.

#100 If I have an excess amount of heavy metals in my urine, will insurance pay for my treatment?

It is possible that insurance companies might cover chelation treatments if a large amount of heavy metals is detected in the urine. Even a small amount of these metals may be harmful. However, the level of heavy metals that is detected is rarely enough to be defined as "heavy metal toxicity" according to industrial standards. It will be nice eventually when EDTA Chelation Therapy is covered by most insurance companies. Most physicians do not want to spend huge efforts to convince insurance companies that an industrial level of heavy metal toxicity exists because this is usually fruitless. Dr. Elmer Cranton has stated that he prefers to spend his primary energies in getting his patients well, not in fighting a legal battle. I agree with Dr. Cranton. My main efforts to get EDTA covered by insurance are directed toward doing research in proving that EDTA is an effective therapy for vascular disease, so that it can be widely used to the benefit of humankind.

Appendix I

The Correlation Between EDTA Chelation Therapy and Improvement in Cardiovascular Function: A Meta-Analysis

by
L. Terry Chappell, M.D., and John P. Stahl, Ph.D.

Published in
Journal of Advancement in Medicine
Volume 6, Number 3, Fall 1993

ABSTRACT: In order to establish whether there is value in treating cardiovascular disease with intravenous EDTA chelation therapy, a meta-analysis was done, based on currently available scientific literature. A thorough literature search identified 40 articles on the subject. Nineteen studies met the criteria for inclusion with data on 22,765 patients. The meta-analysis revealed a correlation coefficient of 0.88, which indicates a high positive relationship between EDTA therapy and improved cardiovascular function. Eighty-seven percent of the patients included in the meta-analysis demonstrated clinical improvement by objective testing.

Introduction

A minority of physicians throughout the world use EDTA chelation therapy to treat atherosclerotic cardiovascular disease. More conventional physicians have from time to time expressed editorial criticism of this treatment, usually claiming that there is little evidence that it is effective.[1-5] Chelating physicians insist that their clinical results are excellent and that attempts to publish their data have been rejected by more widely read and indexed journals.[6-7]

Recently, meta-analysis has emerged as a technique to examine controversial issues in medicine. Experts have proclaimed that it is an effective tool for comparing studies evaluating drugs or medical procedures. Examples include Lau's[8] meta-analysis of therapeutic trials for myocardial infarction and Muldoon's[9] dramatic finding that reduced cholesterol concentrations do not affect overall survival, based on a meta-analysis.

The authors decided to use a meta-analysis to determine the likelihood that EDTA chelation therapy has a positive effect on cardiovascular disease, based on currently available literature.

Techniques for Literature Search

A Medline search revealed that there have been only a few articles published in prominent medical journals. Exerpta Medica, Current Contents, and the French PASCAL databases produced considerably more material. A Science Citation Index search for ten key authors was also performed. Health Periodicals Database and Toxline were scanned. The American College of Advancement in Medicine provided a collection of 80 key articles on the therapeutic use of EDTA.[10] It also offered a substantial volume of abstracts[11] from the world literature on many aspects of the use of chelation therapy. The Journal of Advancement in Medicine has been published since 1987 and has included several important articles on the subject. Since this journal has not been included in the above data bases, individual issues of it were obtained and searched. Finally, individual authors and clinicians were contacted, both to examine their files for additional studies and to provide the raw data from their published studies if it had not been presented in a form needed for the meta-analysis.

Selection of Studies

Criteria were established as follows for the inclusion of studies in the meta-analysis:

1. Limited to human studies;

2. Include only data that specified whether or not the subjects improved;
3. Include only data that referred to objective measurement of improvement in cardiovascular disease.

Because of the strictness of the criteria chosen, many studies were omitted from the meta-analysis. Since the great majority of those omitted showed positive results, it is estimated that inclusion of them would not have significantly changed the outcome of the meta-analysis. However, confidence in the outcome might have been even stronger because of the larger number of studies and subjects considered in the analysis. Numerous animal studies[11,12] show positive effects of EDTA and shed light upon the mechanism of action, but were not included.

A number of important human studies were omitted because they limited their observations to the net statistical change in a group of patients. Although data reported in this form contains much useful information, the studies did not conform to the required criteria. McDonagh, Rudolph and Cheraskin[13] published a collection of 27 articles on the efficacy of EDTA chelation therapy that were originally published in various journals. All but four of them fit this category. One[14] that was included in the meta-analysis because it listed data on individual patients described 30 patients whose carotid artery obstructions were reduced by almost 50 per cent. Riordan and Cheraskin[15,16] published one study on EKG changes and another using the Cornell Medical Index to document clinical change. Guldager and associates[17] in Denmark, a group of cardiovascular surgeons, authored a controversial study in this category that will be discussed in more detail below. The above authors were contacted in an attempt to obtain the raw data on individual patients so that material could be extracted for inclusion in the meta-analysis. Unfortunately, none of the extractions became available in time to be included. Since all these studies were strongly positive except Guldager's, the authors do not feel that they would have impacted the results significantly.

Other reports that contained insufficient data include Robinson's[18] review of 248 patients with various cardiovascular diseases. He commented that the vast majority had symptomatic improvement. Magee[19] mentioned one case treated with EDTA that subsequently required aorto-femoral surgery, but no pre and post testing was offered. Wirebaugh[20] contributed a case report of a patient who improved symptomatically with EDTA but later underwent angioplasty for single vessel disease. The patient did not suffer an infarction, and the only before and after testing listed were negative exercise treadmill tests 5 months after chelation and again after angioplasty. The first case of reversal by chelation of cardiomyopathy due to iron overload was described by Rahko, Salerni, and Uretsky.[21] Deferoxamine instead of EDTA was used as the chelating agent, but both substances remove iron effectively.[22]

Several early papers, especially those by Lamar,[23,24] Clarke and associates[25-28] and Evers,[29] were highly influential because they stimulated many physicians to begin to offer chelation therapy to their patients. These works were omitted because they consisted of large collections of case studies which did not specify objective testing that confirmed that subjects improved with therapy. Olwin and associates[30] and Langhof and associates[31] made general observations, particularly about plasma lipids.

Articles or parts of articles that referred to other chronic degenerative diseases such as scleroderma, Parkinson's disease, osteoporosis, chronic obstructive pulmonary disease, cancer, porphyria and Alzheimer's disease were omitted. More difficult to assess were several articles each on digitalis-induced arrhythmias[32] and reduced left ventricular ejection fraction in Thalassemia Major,[33] both of which were treated successfully with EDTA chelation. These were not included because there were extraneous causes for the cardiovascular problems. A summary of the articles that pertained to EDTA chelation therapy and cardiovascular disease, but were not included in the meta-analysis, is contained in Table 1.

The authors were able to find references to six double- or single-blind studies with controls. All present certain problems. The most reliable appears to be the single-blind cross-over study of 10 patients by Olszewer and Carter.[34] Because the differences between the EDTA treated patients and those who received placebos were so dramatic, the code was broken early and both groups were treated with EDTA. This was ethically the correct step to take, but the study has somewhat less statistical significance because of the atypical design.

Sloth-Nielsen and associates[35] and Guldager and associates[17] published two papers in separate journals on the same clinical trial showing no significant improvement in peripheral vascular patients treated with EDTA. The first paper selected 30 patients who were given angiograms and transcutaneous oxygen tension measurements before, during and after treatment. Twenty-nine of the patients were smokers. The second paper reported on the mean walking distance of all 153 patients, half of whom were given a placebo. Seventy percent of the subjects were smokers and continued to smoke. Three critiques of these papers[36-38] have been published, based on interviews of patients and nurses who participated in the study. It is contended by Cranton and Frackelton that smokers were deliberately chosen to be subjects and patients were instructed to take iron-containing tablets during the treatment period, both of which would tend to lessen the benefits of EDTA considerably. They also state that the study was not blind as claimed, that pain at the IV site was not as expected and that some patients who claimed to be better were placed in the category of no improvement. Although these allegations are disturbing, judgment is not made on them at this time. Further observations reveal that the study involved very sick patients with A/B indices averaging 0.5, limited treatment (20 IVs), and the omission of intravenous magnesium from the standard protocol. Patients receiving EDTA improved more than placebo treated patients in both walking distance and A/B index at 6 months followup, but the results were not statistically significant. According to the criteria, the first paper is included in the meta-analysis because it reports results for individual patients. The second is omitted because the data needed on the individual patients for this study were not available.

Olszewer and Carter refer to a double-blind study done at the University of Heidelberg in Germany by Diehm.[39] The study compared intravenous EDTA to benzcyclan (a vasoactive drug that is also an anticoagulant) in the treatment of peripheral vascular disease for 45 patients. Both groups improved by 70-76 percent in walking distance, although three months after treatment, the EDTA group reported a greater improvement. The author concluded that the improvement was a "placebo effect," even though no placebo was used. Olszewer and Carter[40] stated that the raw data revealed that four patients treated with EDTA experienced more than a 1000-meter increase in walking distance but were excluded from the statistical analysis as outliers. It was also shown that 7 out of 10 patients with gangrene made satisfactory recoveries with EDTA chelation therapy. Since the paper itself did not reveal data on individual patients, it was not included in this meta-analysis.

A double-blind study of a small sample of patients was apparently completed at Baylor University School of Medicine several years ago, but the results have not yet been published, and the raw data were not obtainable. Foundation Partners, Inc. is the holder of an Investigational New Drug permit issued by the Food and Drug Administration and is co-sponsor of a FDA approved, double-blind study of EDTA treatment of vascular disease. Martin Rubin and Ross Gordon were instrumental in designing and working out the specifics of this study, which has not yet been completed. Another ongoing study by Van Rij in New Zealand is nearing completion. None of these studies were available for the meta-analysis.

Hoekstra, Gedye, Scarchilli, Parente and associates[41] have completed a large retrospective study of 19,147 patients utilizing thermography pre and post EDTA treatment for peripheral vascular disease. In spite of its being unpublished, the so-called Cypher study has been allowed as evidence in several legal proceedings and was instrumental in obtaining government acceptance of the treatment in New Zealand. The authors allowed use of the pre-publication draft of their paper for this meta-analysis. All patients had at least moderate stenosis and 86 percent of them showed measurable improvement after treatment with EDTA. A control group of 64 patients did not improve. The statistician conducted a blinded re-analysis of the data for a representative sample, which confirmed the results.

There is no question that the Kitchell and Meltzer study[42] should be a part of the meta-analysis. Since the data from two earlier studies are included in their "re-appraisal" article, which was instrumental in discouraging further research for almost two decades, the updated information in that article was used. Of note, as pointed out by Cranston and Frackelton,[7] the data showed positive results with some very sick patients, despite the title of the article.

Another study that qualified for this meta-analysis was that by Olszewer and Carter,[40] which reported on 2482 patients that fit the criteria. Other patients in this study were omitted because they were not cardiovascular patients. Clarke and associates[25] provided the initial observations on EDTA for vascular problems in 1955. One of their follow-up papers[43] discussed objective data on individual patients. Casdorph[44,45] with two articles by himself and one with Farr[46] made significant contributions in the '80s. Godfrey[47] listed 27 patients in a letter to the New Zealand Medical Journal. Case studies by Morgan[48] and Brucknerova[49] met the criteria. Hancke and Flytlie[50] of Denmark provided EDTA chelation for patients who were on the waiting list for bypass or amputation, with the impressive results that 58 out of 65 bypass candidates and 24 out of 27 amputation candidates were able to cancel their surgery. In the same paper, which was reported at two European medical meetings, they described a larger series of coronary artery disease patients whose ST segments improved on exercise EKGs and peripheral vascular patients whose walking distances and ankle/brachial indices showed consistent gains with treatment. They also recorded symptomatic relief in as many as 92 percent of CAD patients, but the latter was excluded from the analysis because it was subjective. Their data were available but have not yet been published. The four studies that were included in the meta-analysis by McDonagh, Rudolph and Cheraskin[14,51-53] utilized doppler ultrasound, oculocerebrovascular analysis and the A/B index to document improvement in carotid and peripheral circulation after treatment. McGillem and associates[4] provided a case report of a patient with severe coronary artery disease

Table 1

STUDIES LINKING EDTA WITH CARDIOVASCULAR DISEASE NOT USED IN META-ANALYSIS

AUTHOR	JOURNAL & DATE	DIAGNOSIS	TEST	NO. OF SUBJECTS	RESULTS
McDonagh, et al	Med Hyp/81	Hyperlipidemia	Cholesterol	221	Chol reduced ave of 25-31 points
McDonagh, et al	Med Hyp/82	Hyperlipidemia	Chol/HDL Ratio	358	Low ratios rise, high ratios fall
McDonagh, et al	J Ortho Pys/82	CAD/Fatigue	Cornell MedIndex	95	Fatigue scores imprvd by 39%
Cheraskin, et al	Jofl AP Med/84	CAD	HR w/ SEKG	50	HR decreased by 8.7 to 9.2%
McDonagh, et al	J Ortho Pys/85	Pts w/Chronic Dis	Cornell MedIndex	139	Symptoms scores red. by 13-31%
Riordan, et al	J Ortho Med/89	Hypertension	Cornell MedIndex	28	23% symptom reduction
Riordan, et al	J Adv Med/88	Elev Lead Levels	QRS Interval	28	Reduced interval .07 to .064
Lamar	J Am Ger Soc/66	CAD, PVD, CVD	Non-Inv Vasc Test/Symptoms	53	Marked imprvmt, dementia and vision better
Lamar	Angiology/64	PVD, CAD, DM	Symptoms Decr Insulin	15	All improved, insulin red. in 7
Boyle, Clarke	Fed Proc/61	CAD, Angina	Symptoms/ EKG	10	9 Improved, sev had better EKG's
Clarke, et al	A J Med Sci/55	Angina, PVD	Symptoms	22	Unusual symptoms relief/hearing imp
Clarke, et al	A J Med Sci/60	CAD	Symptoms	76	96% improved
Clarke, et al		Interm Claudic	Symptoms	31	87% improved
Clarke, et al		CVD	Symptoms	25	100% improved
Clarke	A M J Card/60	PVD, CAD, CVD	Symptoms	Several Hundred	>87% improved incr. WD, decr Mort
Robinson	N Z Med J/82	CAD, PVD, HBP	EKG/BP, Pain	248	Pain relieved, BP & EKG's better
Evers	ACAM/79	CAD, CVD, PVD	Symptoms w/dist	3,000	> 90% Improved
Olwin, et al	Soc Exp Biol/68	Hyperlipidemia	Plasma Lipids	34	Lipids lowered, esp. trigl.
Langhof	Proc Angiol/61	PVD, High Chol	Symptoms/ Chol	12	Sympt. improved, Chol lowered
Hancke, et al	-/93	CAD	Working Capac	208	84% Improved
Hancke, et al			Angina Sympt	162	91% Improved
Hancke, et al			NTG Demand	133	92% Improved
Guldager, et al	J Int Med/92	Severe PVD	WD, A/B Index	66	EDTA pts imprv more than placebo group, but diff not statistically significant
Magee	Med J Aust/85	PVD	Need for Surg	1	Failed treatment
Wirebaugh, et al	DICP An Ph/90	CAD	Need for Angiopl	1	Failed treatment
Rahko, et al	J A Coll Card/86	cardiomyop	Symptoms	1	Recovered - DFO, not EDTA
Diehm	Z Deut Herz/86	PVD	W Dist	24	Both EDTA & Bncy impr 70-76% EDTA was better at 3 mos. Not statistically significant

and renal problems that received low dose EDTA and failed to show improvement in his angiograms post-treatment. Van der Schaar,[54] who is a cardiovascular surgeon from the Netherlands, conducted a particularly interesting calculation of the double and triple product to demonstrate increased exercise tolerance in chelated patients. The studies that were included in the meta-analysis are listed in Table 2.

Method of Analysis

The greater part of available research concerning the effect of EDTA chelation therapy on cardiovascular disease is of the pretest-posttest, without a control group, design. With this type of study the investigator measures the cardiovascular capability of each patient in a group before treatment, applies the treatment to each member of the group, and then measures the cardiovascular capability of each member of the group after treatment. The pretest-posttest data are then tabulated in some papers with statistical analysis, sometimes without.

Because of the lack of placebo controlled studies performed by researchers using EDTA chelation therapy, the efficacy of this technique has not spread widely into the medical community. To maintain scientific objectivity physicians require significant evidence that therapeutic efficacy exists before adopting any questionable therapy for use in their individual practice, and rightly so. Even though placebo control has, for the most part, been absent in existing EDTA studies, this does not mean that the data collected are not valid or useful. When a treatment effect is actually present, then the data used in a properly designed meta-analysis will show the presence and size of the effect whether the studies used are placebo controlled double-blind studies, or are pretest-posttest studies without control groups. This assumes, of course, that good design and measuring techniques are used and that the variables are not confounded.

Since significant statistical verification of the efficacy of EDTA therapy has not been demonstrated in many reports in the existing literature, this meta-analysis will use existing study data to provide this evidence. The procedure chosen is to determine the extent of the relationship, the "effect size," between EDTA chelation therapy and cardiovascular improvement. The correlation coefficient is the statistical descriptor selected for this meta-analysis because it indicates the degree of relationship between two variables. A correlation coefficient of 0.0 would indicate that there is no relationship between EDTA chelation therapy and improvement in cardiovascular capability, while a value of 1.0 would indicate a perfect relationship between the two variables. Variables with correlation coefficients greater than 0.7 are considered to be strongly related.

There are two variables considered in this analysis: the method of treatment and the degree of improvement. Additionally, these two variables are conditioned to be discrete dichotomies. The method of treatment variable then is limited to the values, EDTA chelation therapy vs. no therapy and the degree of improvement variable is limited to the values of significant cardiovascular improvement vs. no improvement or worse. Formulating the variables in this way allows for the calculation of the phi (ϕ) coefficient, a special case of the Pearson r correlation coefficient when both variables are discrete dichotomies.[55] After the phi (ϕ) correlation coefficients are calculated for the individual studies, the overall result of the meta-analysis is determined. The composite ϕ is a synthesis of the results of each of the individual studies. It is formulated by calculating a weighted average correlation coefficient where each individual study correlation used is weighted by the number of patients in the particular study.[56]

Table 2
Data From Unpublished Studies Used in Meta-Analysis

DOCTOR	LOCATION	DIAGNOSES	OBJECTIVE TEST	SUBJECTS	IMPROVED	SAME/WORSE
Garg	London, England	ASHD, PVD, CAROTID INSUFFICIENCY	ANGIOGRAM (15), DOPPLERS (31)	32	31	1
Hart	Spokane, WA (USA)	PVD, CAD, CVD, HBP	DOPPLER, EKG, CHOL, WDIST	7	7	0
Hodara	Brazil	CAD, CVD	EKG, ULTRASOUND	1	1	0
Janson	Cambridge, MA (USA)	CAD	CHOL, TRIG, NEED FOR MED	10	7	3
Laird	Leichester, NC (USA)	PVD	DOPPLER	19	12	7
Affandi	Indonesia	CAD, CVD	SEKG, EKG, EMG, BP, CHOL	10	10	0
Bock	Rhinebeck, NY (USA)	PVD, CAD, CVD	SEKG, EKG, DOPLR, CARTID ULTRASOUND	11	10	1
Born	Grand Rapids, MI (USA)	CAD, PVD, CVD	DOPPLER, EKG, CARDIOINTEGRAPH	748	645	103
Darbro	Indianapolis, IN (USA)	ASHD	SMAC 24	10	10	0
Goldberg	Dayton, OH (USA)	CAD, HYPERLIPIDEMIA	CHOL, TRIG, REPEAT BYPASS	4	3	1
Gonzalez	Homosassa, FL (USA)	CAD, PVD	SEKG, DOPPLER, CHOL	3	3	0
Gunter	Camilla, GA (USA)	PVD, CAD, CVD	DOPPLER	7	6	1
Eckerly, Dole	Plymouth, MN (USA)	PVD, CAD, CVD, HBP	DOPPLER, BP, COGNITIVE FUNCTION	19	19	0
Harris	Island Heights NJ (USA)	GANGRENE	HEALED	1	1	0
Maulfair	Mertztown, PA (USA)	PVD, RAYNAUD'S CAD, CVD	DOPPLER, SEKG	9	8	1
Penwell	Linden, MI (USA)	CAD (21), CVD (3), PVD (25)	HM, EKG, SEKG, DOPPLER, XSURG	49	42	7
Reynoso	Manila	CAD, PVD	CATH (3), DOPPLER	8	8	0
Chappell	Bluffton, OH (USA)	PVD, CVD	DOPPLER	33	27	6
Sams	Columbus, MS (USA)	CVD, PVD	DOPPLER	18	18	0
Magaziner	Cherry Hill, NJ (USA)	CVD	CAROTID ULTRASOUND	1	1	0
Speckhart	Norfolk, VA (USA)	CAD	STRESS THALIUM	1	1	0
Young	Salem, OR (USA)	CVD, CAD, PVD	DOPPLER, HOLTER, EKG, CHOL	35	32	3
Braverman	Skillman, NJ (USA)	CAD	PET SCAN	1	1	0
Rozema	Landrum, SC (USA)	PVD	DOPPLER	53	50	3
Kindness	Bluffton, OH (USA)	HYPERLIPIDEMIA	APOLIPOPROTEINS	29	26	3
DeSousa	Brazil	CAD, PVD, CVD, HBP	ANGIOGRAMS (3), EKG, DOPPLER	9	9	0
Moharram	Santa Barbara CA (USA)	CAD	BYPASS NEEDED	1	1	0
Olzsewer, et al	Brazil	CAD	SEKG	30	26	4
Godfrey	New Zealand	PVD, CAD	DOPPLER, SEKG, MEDS NEEDED	16	16	0
Levin	New York, NY (USA)	CAD, PVD, CVD	SEKG, HM, EKG, PVR, DOPPLER	22	15	7
Wolverton	Clarksville, IN (USA)	PVD, CAD, CVD	ANGIOGRAM (2) SEKG, EKG, DOPPLER	21	19	2
Walker	St. Louis, MO (USA)	CAD, CVD	CAROTID ULTRASOUND, ACTIVITY TOLERATED	23	21	2
			TOTALS	1241	1086 (88%)	155 (12%)

Calculation of the phi (φ) correlation coefficient, as described for each individual study, implies that each study included in the meta-analysis was conducted in the following manner. The study subjects were pretested for some aspect of cardiovascular capacity. The treatment group was then treated with EDTA chelation therapy while treatment was withheld from an assumed control group. Both groups, the treatment group and the assumed control group, were then posttested on the same aspect of cardiovascular capacity. Sufficient data then exists to construct the 2 x 2 contingency table used for computing the phi (φ) correlation coefficient for that particular study.

Glass, McGaw and Smith[69] in their section on Studies Without Control Groups suggest that traditional or baseline values can be used as a "control" condition. They indicate that "experiments often have no untreated control' condition" but that "a control condition of no treatment can be defined and included." For the purpose of this meta-analysis, then, simply consider the existing study data to be the data for the treatment group and compare the improvement in cardiovascular function of the treatment group to a control group defined to have no improvement in cardiovascular capability.

It needs to be shown that the assumption of a no-treatment control group with no improvement is reasonable. This meta-analysis will use the blinded study by Olszewer, Sabbag and Carter[34] to show this. Their study is of particular interest to this meta-analytic procedure because the code was broken and as a consequence the data is in a particularly useful form. The specific data of interest are contained in Table 3 Blood Pressure Index of their paper, and are partially reproduced below.

	Group Assigned to EDTA			Group Assigned to Placebo		
	Baseline	10 EDTA	20 EDTA	Baseline	10 Placebo	10 Placebo/ 10 EDTA
Rest	0.66	0.89	0.95	0.62	0.63	0.86
Exercise	0.54	0.78	0.88	0.56	0.54	0.75

To construct the contingency table a control group was hypothesized where the no-treatment control group was equal in size and other characteristics with the treatment group. It was assumed that there is no improvement with no treatment and data will be entered into the table to that effect. This may or may not be true. It is entirely possible that there might be improvement within the control group, even though treatment has been withheld. Some studies are more likely than others to show an improvement for no treatment. An examination of the Olszewer, Sabbag and Carter data[34] indicates that there was essentially no change in placebo subject function whereas there was a significant change in EDTA subject function over 10 treatments. This can indicate one of two possibilities; either the placebo is having no effect or the placebo-treated subjects might not be responding to any treatment, either placebo or EDTA. The second scenario is rejected because the response of the placebo subjects showed an improvement when EDTA was substituted for the placebo for the remaining 10 infusions. Therefore, it is concluded that for similar populations using the EDTA chelation therapy protocol the assumption of a no-improvement control group is valid.

As an example, suppose that a particular study indicates that 15 out of 20 patients had evidence of a significant improvement in cardiovascular capability after the EDTA treatment protocol while 5 patients showed no improvement. Note that for the "no treatment" or "control" group the posttest value equals the pretest value for "no improvement" and the corresponding table entries are thus (0,20). For the "treatment" group it is clear that the table entries are (15,5). The 2 x 2 contingency table and corresponding ϕ correlation coefficient is given below.

	Improvement	No Improvement	TOTALS
Control (No Treatment)	0	20	20
EDTA Treatment	15	5	20
TOTALS	15	25	40

The ϕ correlation coefficient calculation is:

$$\phi = \frac{(15)(20) - (0)(5)}{[(20 + 0)(15 + 5)(0 + 25)(20 + 5)]^{\frac{1}{2}}} = 0.77$$

which indicates a high correlation. With a high correlation it can be stated that there is a positive relationship between EDTA chelation therapy and improvement in cardiovascular function. Traditionally, the square of the coefficient of correlation or the coefficient of determination is used as an estimate of the shared variance between the two variables.[57]

For correlation interpreting purposes Table 3 can be used as a guide.

TABLE 3			
Group Size	Improvement	No Improvement	ϕ
20	20	0	1.00
20	15	5	0.77
20	5	15	0.38
20	0	20	0.00

Hinkle, Wiersma and Jurs[55] provide guidelines for interpreting the size of a correlation coefficient, which are listed in Table 4.

Table 4	
INTERPRETING THE SIZE OF A CORRELATION COEFFICIENT (HINKLE, WIERSMA & JURS)	
.90 to 1.00	Very high positive correlation
.70 to .90	High positive correlation
.50 to .70	Moderate positive correlation
.30 to .50	Low positive correlation
.00 to .30	Little if any correlation

Table 5

CORRELATION COEFFICIENT FOR ALL STUDIES

AUTHOR	SUBJECTS	IMPROVED	SAME/WORSE	CORRELATION
Olszewer, Carter	2,482	2,379	103	0.96
Clarke	20	19	1	0.95
Kitchell, et al	38	23	15	0.66
Sloth-Nielson	30	2	28	0.19
Casdorph	15	14	1	0.94
Casdorph, Farr	4	4	0	1.00
Casdorph	18	17	1	0.95
Olszewer, Carter	10	10	0	1.00
Godfrey	27	25	2	0.93
Morgan	2	2	0	1.00
Brucknerova	2	2	0	1.00
Hancke	92	82	10	0.90
Hancke	253	175	78	0.73
Hancke	308	272	36	0.89
McGillem	1	0	1	0.00
Rudolph, McDonagh	1	1	0	1.00
McDonagh, et al	57	50	7	0.88
McDonagh, et al	117	95	22	0.83
Hoekstra, et al	19,147	16,466	2,681	0.87
Van der Schaar	111	111	0	1.00
Rudolph, et al	30	30	0	1.00

OVERALL CORRELATION COEFFICIENT = 0.88

The following formula is used to calculate a composite correlation coefficient. The i_{th} study has N_i subjects with correlation coefficient-$_i$. The composite correlation, ϕ composite represents the relationship between improvement in cardiovascular activity and EDTA chelation therapy taking data from all of the studies into account. The effect of each individual study is weighted by the number of patients in the study. A 10-subject study has about 1/10th the weight of a 100-subject study.

$$\Phi \text{ composite} = \frac{\sum N_i \Phi_i}{\sum N_i}$$

Results

Table 5 (left) shows those studies included in the meta-analysis, indicating the individual correlation coefficient for each study and the overall correlation coefficient. The overall correlation coefficient is equal to 0.88. This value indicates a highly positive correlation between EDTA chelation therapy and improvement in cardiovascular function. The traditional interpretation of using the square of the correlation coefficient as an estimate of the variability between the two variables indicates that approximately 77 percent of the variability in improvement in cardiovascular function is associated with the treatment of EDTA chelation therapy.

The remaining 23 percent is associated with other unknown factors. Wolfe[56] indicates that Rosenthal and Rubin provide an alternate "insightful" way to appraise the significance of correlation coefficients with their "binomial effect size display" (BESD) for 2 x 2 contingency tables. For our variables, the BESD is the estimated difference in success rate between the two variables, EDTA chelation therapy and improvement in cardiovascular function. That is, for a correlation coefficient of 0.88 we would expect an increase of success in cardiovascular improvement from 6 percent of patients improved with no treatment to 94 percent of patients improved as a result of applying EDTA chelation therapy. The Binomial Effect Size Display illustrating this condition is shown in Table 6. Note that the correlation coefficient calculated or the data of this table is .88. The formula used for calculating the success rate is:

Success Rate $\pm$ .50 ϕ / 2

Table 6			
	Improvement	No Improvement	TOTALS
Control (No Treatment)	6	94	100
EDTA Treatment	94	6	100
TOTALS	100	100	200

Tables 7 and 8 demonstrate that there is little difference in the correlation coefficient whether the analysis is limited to large studies or small studies.

Table 7
Small Studies Only

AUTHOR	SUBJECTS	IMPROVED	SAME/WORSE	CORRELATION
Clarke	20	19	1	0.95
Kitchell, et al	38	23	15	0.66
Sloth-Nielson	30	2	28	0.19
Casdorph	15	14	1	0.94
Casdorph, Farr	4	4	0	1.00
Casdorph	18	17	1	0.95
Olszewer, Carter	10	10	0	1.00
Godfrey	27	25	2	0.93
Morgan	2	2	0	1.00
Brucknerova	2	2	0	1.00
Hancke	92	82	10	0.90
Hancke	253	175	78	0.73
Hancke	308	272	36	0.89
McGillem	1	0	1	0.00
Rudolph, McDonagh	1	1	0	1.00
McDonagh, et al	57	50	7	0.88
McDonagh, et al	117	95	22	0.83
Van der Schaar	111	111	0	1.00
Rudolph, et al	30	30	0	1.00

OVERALL CORRELATION COEFFICIENT = 0.84

Table 8
Large Studies Only

AUTHOR	SUBJECTS	IMPROVED	SAME/WORSE	CORRELATION
Olszewer, Carter	2,482	2,379	103	0.96
Hoekstra, et al	19,147	16,466	2,681	0.87

OVERALL CORRELATION COEFFICIENT = 0.88

Mechanism of Action

Gordon and Vance,[58] Halstead[59] and Cranton and Frackelton[7] have reviewed the pharmacology of EDTA in the treatment of cardiovascular disease. Emphasis was placed[7] on reduction of free radicals by removing heavy metals, iron and copper and by antioxidant activity. Bjorksten[60] suggest that chelation might be valuable in life extension. Deucher[61] described chelation as an "antioxidant strategy," and Gutteridge[62] identified increased effectiveness of hydroxyl-radical scavengers in the presence of EDTA. An editorial by Zylke[63] mentioned edetic acid (EDTA) as a possible treatment to control oxygen radicals. Kaman, Rudolph, McDonagh and Walker[64] demonstrated the removal of metastatic calcium in rabbit aortas. Kindness and Frackelton[65] showed the beneficial therapeutic effects of EDTA chelation of inhibiting platelet aggregation and prolonging the partial thromboplastin time. Lamb and Leuke[66] recently discussed the concentration required in vitro for EDTA to inhibit the oxidation of LDL by macrophages and by copper. An excellent compendium of articles, including the protocol recommended by the American College for Advancement in Medicine for EDTA administration, was published in *A Textbook of EDTA Chelation Therapy* in 1989.[67]

Discussion

Lugo-Miro and associates[68] suggested that meta-analysis is one of the best tools to evaluate controversial therapies. This paper has utilized a similar technique to estimate the statistical relationship between EDTA chelation therapy and the positive effect that the therapy has on atherosclerotic cardiovascular disease. The results show a high positive correlation, indicating its efficacy.

More than 40 published reports and two unpublished studies have been examined in this paper. Only one multi-patient study,[35] which was conducted by Danish vascular surgeons, contained data that showed negative results. The trials by Diehm[38] and Kitchell and associates[42] both demonstrated favorable clinical outcomes, in spite of negative conclusions. Nineteen studies met the criteria and were included in the analysis. The meta-analysis thus contained results from the treatment of 22,765 patients, 87 percent of whom had favorable outcomes. This percentage is changed very little whether the large studies by Olszewer and Carter and by Hoekstra and associates are included or not.

Only those improvements measurable by an objective test were accepted as evidence of a favorable outcome. Those patients who improved clinically but did not improve their objective test results were placed in the category of the same or worse.

One problem with assessing therapeutic modalities is that negative data are sometimes not published. Glass, McGaw and Smith[69] indicate that the selection of papers may bias a meta-analysis. To minimize this bias potential, the authors are in the process of collecting additional data.

The majority of studies considered functional assessments of the patients. Sloth-Nielson and associates[35] relied on arteriograms, which may have ignored improvements in small vessel blood flow. Several studies demonstrated that maximal improvement with EDTA therapy occurred up to three months or more after the basic course of therapy was completed. Reasons for this effect are unknown. Possible explanations include a delayed antioxidant effect, a gradual restoration of depleted trace minerals or that causative metals, acting as free radical catalysts, are removed, thus allowing a natural healing process to occur over time.

The safety of EDTA treatment has been acknowledged by the FDA in the Foundation Partners trial, and no further studies were required to demonstrate safety under the IND. Our literature search revealed no significant concerns for safety, as long as the published protocol[67] is carefully followed. Reports of toxicity[70,71] involved the rapid daily administration of a much higher dose of EDTA than is allowed in the protocol.

In 1984, the American College of Advancement in Medicine estimated that 400,000 patients had been treated by member physicians with no fatalities attributed to the recommended protocol.[72] The number of patients treated safely has probably doubled since that time.

Recently, the Great Lakes Association of Clinical Medicine released a white paper on The Cost Effectiveness of Alternative Medicine in the Workplace.[73] The chapter on EDTA chelation made a case for the consideration of this therapy as an alternative or adjunct to bypass surgery and angioplasty as a cost saving measure.

Conclusion

This meta-analysis offers very strong evidence that EDTA is effective in the treatment of cardiovascular disease. A number of studies are in the planning stage, but have not been activated for lack of financial support. The authors hope that this statistically significant meta-analysis might speed this support. Interest is growing in New Zealand, Canada, Great Britain, Denmark, Brazil and other countries. EDTA therapy needs to assume its place in the treatment of cardiovascular disease.

Acknowledgements

The authors extend their appreciation for the support given by many individuals in the preparation of this paper. We are particularly indebted to Professor Ronald L. Evans, Department of Mathematics, Ohio Northern University for his statistical contribution to the preparation of the meta-analysis, and to Mark Wettler, Karen Slessor and Sara Bassitt for their help in searching the literature.

References

1. Editorial: Diagnostic and therapeutic technology assessment: chelation therapy. JAMA 1983; 250-672.

2. Editorial: EDTA chelation therapy for arteriosclerotic heart disease. Med Lett Drugs Ther 1981; 23:51.

3. Soffer A. Chelation therapy for arteriosclerosis. JAMA 1975; 233:1206-1207.

4. McGillem MJ, Mancini GBJ. Inefficacy of EDTA chelation therapy for atherosclerosis. NEJM 1988; 318:1618-1619.

5. Patterson R. Chelation therapy and Uncle John. Can Med As J 1989; 40:829-831.

6. Cranton EM. The current status of EDTA chelation therapy. J Hol Med 1985; 7:3-7.

7. Cranton EM, Frackelton JP. Free radical pathology in age-associated diseases; treatment with EDTA chelation, nutrition and antioxidants. J Hol Med 1984; 6:6-37.

8. Lau J, Antman EM, Jimenez-Silva J, Kupelnick B. Cumulative meta-analysis of therapeutic trials for myocardial infarctioin. N Engl J Med 1992; 327:248-255.

9. Muldoon MF, Manuck SB, Matthews KA. Lowering cholesterol concentrations and mortality: a quantitative review of primary intervention trials. Br Med J 1990; 301:309-314.

10. Chelation bibliography—a collection of 80 articles. American College for Advancement in Medicine, 23121 Verdugo Drive, Suite 204, Laguna Hills, CA 92653, 1979.

11. ACAM compilation of EDTA abstracts and references. American College for Advancement in Medicine, 23121 Verdugo Drive, Suite 204, Laguna Hills, CA 92653, 1990.

12. Uhl HS, Dysko RC, St. Clair RW, EDTA reduces liver cholesterol content in cholesterol fed rabbits. Atherosclerosis 1992; 96:181-188.

13. McDonagh EW, Rudolph CJ. A collection of published papers showing the efficacy of EDTA chelation therapy. McDonagh Medical Center, Gladstone, MO. 1989.

14. Rudolph CJ, McDonagh EW, Barbar RK. A non-surgical approach to obstructive carotid atheromatous stenosis: and independent study. J Adv Med 1991; 4:157-166.

15. Riordan HD, Cheraskin E, Dirks M, et al. EDTA treatment of intermittent claudication—a double-blind, placebo controlled study. J Int Med 1992; 231: 261-267.

16. Riordan HD, Cheraskin E, Dirks M, et al. EDTA chelation/hypertension study: clinical patterns as judged by the Cornell Medical Index questionaire. J Ortho Med 1989; 4:91-95.

17. Guldager B, Jelnes R, Jorgensen SJ, et al. EDTA treatment of intermittent claudication—a double-blind, placebo-controlled study. J Int Med 1992; 231: 261-267.

18. Robinson DM, chelation therapy. NZ Med J 1982; 95: 750.

19. Magee HR. Reply to Gibson TJB: Chelation therapy for atherosclerosis. Med J. Aust 1985; 143: 127.

20. Wirebaugh SR, Geracts DR. Apparent failure of edetic acid chelation therapy for the treatment of coronary atherosclerosis. DICP Ann Ph 1990; 24:22-25.

21. Rahko, PS, Calerni R. Uretsky BF. Successful reversal by chelation therapy of congestive cardiomyopathy due to iron overload. J Am Coll Card 1986; 8:436-440.

22. Rudolph CJ, McDonagh EW, Barber RK. Effect of EDTA chelation on serum iron. J Adv Med 1991; 4:39-45.

23. Lamar CP. Chelation endarterectomy for occlusive atherosclerosis. J Am Ger Soc 1966; 14:272-294.

24. Lamar CP. Chelation therapy of occlusive arteriosclerosis in diabetic patients. Angiology 1964; 15:379-394.

25. Clarke NE, Clarke CN, Mosher RE. The "in vivo" dissolution of metastatic calcium: an approach to atherosclerosis. Am J Med Sci 1955; 229:142-149.

26. Clarke NE. Arteriosclerosis, occlusive vascular disease and EDTA. Am J Cardiology 1960; 2:233-236.

27. Clarke NE. Treatment of occlusive vascular disease with disodium ethylene diamine tetraacetic acid (EDTA). AmJ Med Sci 1960 June: 732-744.

28. Boyle AJ, Clarke NE, Mosher RE, McCann DS. Chelation therapy in circulatory and sclerosing diseases. Fed Proc 1961; 29:243-251.

29. Evers R. Chelation of vascular atheromatous disease (experience with 3000 patients). Private communication 1975; see ref. 10.

30. Olwin JH, Koppel JR. Reduction of elevated plasma lipid levels in atherosclerosis following EDTA therapy. Soc Exp Biol & Med Proc 1968; 128:1137-1140.

31. Langhof H, Zanbel H. Voelkner E. Treatment of arteriosclerosis with Na ethylenediaminetetraacetate (EDTA). metab Parietis Vasorum, Papers Intern Congr Angiol 5th 1961; 1021-1024.

32. Surawicz B, MacDonald MG, Kaljot V, Bettinger JC. Treatment of cardiac arrhythmias with salts of ethylenediamine tetraacetic acid. Am Heart J 1959; 58:493-503.

33. Lerner N, Blei F, Bierman F, Johnson L. Chelation therapy and cardiac status in older patients with thalassemia major. Am J Ped Hem Onc 1990; 12:56-60.

34. Olszewer E, Sabbag, FC, Carter JP. A pilot double-blind study of sodium-magnesium EDTA in peripheral vascular disease. J Nat Med As 1990; 82:173-177.

35. Sloth-Nielsen J, Guldager B, Mouritzen C, et al. Arteriographic findings in EDTA chelation therapy on peripheral arteriosclerosis. Am J Surg 1991; 162:122-125.

36. Editorial: EDTA chelation: a rebuttal. J Adv Med 1992; 5:3-5.

37. Cranton EM, Frackelton JP. Negative Danish study of EDTA chelation biased. Townsend Letter for Doctors 1992 July:604-605.

38. Hancke C, Flytlie K. Manipulation with EDTA. Ugeskar Laegar 1992; 154:2213-2215.

39. Diehm C. "Wonder remedy chelation" — Claims and actuality. Zeitschrift der Deutschen Herzstiftung 1986; 10:11-15.

40. Olszewer E, Carter JP. EDTA chelation therapy in chronic degenerative disease Med Hypoth 1988; 27:41-49.

41. Hoekstra PP III, Gedye JL, Hoekstra P, et al. Serial infusions of magnesium disodium ethylene diamine tetraacetic acid enhance perfusion in human extremities. Pre-publication draft. Therma-Scan, Inc. 26711 Woodward Ave, Huntington Woods, MI 48070, 1993.

42. Kitchell JR, Palmon F, Aytan N, Meltzer L. The treatment of coronary artery disease with disodium EDTA: a reappraisal. Am J Cardiol 1963; 11:501-506.

43. Clarke NE, Clarke C, Mosher R. Treatment of angina pectoris with disodium ethylene tetraacetic acid. Am J. Med Sci 1956 Dec:654-666.

44. Casdorph HR. EDTA chelation therapy, efficacy in arteriosclerotic heart disease. J Hol Med 1981; 3:53-59.

45. Casdorph HR. EDTA chelation therapy II, efficacy in brain disorders. J Hol Med 1981; 3:101-117.

46. Casdorph HR, Farr CH. EDTA chelation therapy III, treatment of peripheral arterial occlusion, an alternative to amputation. J Hol Med 1983; 5:3-15.

47. Godfrey ME, EDTA chelation as a treatment of arteriosclerosis. NZ Med J 1990; 103:162-163.

48. Morgan K. Myocardial ischemia treated with nutrients and intravenous EDTA chelation. Report of two cases. J Adv Med 1991; 4:47-56.

49. Brucknerova O, Malinovska V. First clinical experience with combined treatment with chelation III and glucagon in ischaemic disease of the lower extremities. Cas Lek Ces 1980; 119:814-815.

50. Hancke C, Flytlie K. Benefits of EDTA chelation therapy on arteriosclerosis. Pre-publication draft, presented in 1992 in Frankfort, Germany and Milano, Italy. Testcenter Kredslobsklinik, Lyngby Hovegade 17, DK-2800-Lyngby 45 42 88 09 00 (Denmark).

51. Rudolph CJ, McDonagh EW. Effect of EDTA chelation and supportive multi vitamin/trace mineral supplementation on carotid circulation: case report. J Adv Med 1990; 3:5-12.

52. McDonagh EW, Rudolph CJ, Cheraskin E. The effect of EDTA chelation therapy plus multivitamin/trace mineral supplementation upon vascular dynamics (ankle/branchial systolic blood pressure). J Hol Med 1985; 7:16-22.

54. Van der Schaar P. Exercise tolerance in chelation therapy. J Adv Med 1989; 2:563-566.

55. Hinkle DE, Wiersma W, Jurs SG. Applied Statistics for the Behavioral Sciences. Boston, MA, Houghton Mifflin 1979:85-101.

56. Wolf FM. Meta-Analysis Quantitative Methods for Research Synthesis. Newberry Park, CA, Sage Publications 1986:31-33.

57. Scheafler RL, McClave JT. Probability and Statistics for Engineers. Boston, MA, PWS Publishers 1986:363-371.

58. Gordon GB, Vance RB. EDTA chelation therapy for atherosclerosis: history and mechanisms of action. Ost Ann 1976; 4:38-62.

59. Halstead BM. The Scientific Basis of EDTA Chelation Therapy, Colton, California, Golden Quill Publishers 1979.

60. Bjorksten J. Possibilities and limitations of chelation as a means for life extension. J Adv Med 1989; 2:77-78.

61. Deucher DP. EDTA chelation therapy: an antioxidant strategy. J Adv Med 1988; 1:182-190.

62. Gutteridge, JMC. Ferrous-salt-promoted damage to deoxyribose and benzoate, the increased effectiveness of hydroxyl-radical scavengers in the presence of EDTA. Biochem J 1987; 243:709-714.

63. Zylke J. Studying oxygen's life-and-death roles if taken from or reintroduced into tissue. JAMA 1988; 259: 964-965.

64. Kaman RL, Rudolph CJ, McDonagh EW, Walker FM. Effect of EDTA chelation therapy on aortic calcium in rabbits on atherogenic diets: quantitative and histochemical studies. J Adv Med 1990; 3:13-22.

65. Kindness G, Frackelton JP. Effect of ethylene diamine tetraacetic acid (EDTA) on platelet aggregation in human blood. J Adv Med 1989; 2:519-530.

66. Lamb DJ, Leake DS. The effect of EDTA on the oxidation of low density lipoprotein. Atherosclerosis 1992; 94:35-42.

67. Cranton EM; ed: A textbook on EDTA chelation therapy. J Adv Med 1989; 2:1-416.

68. Lugo-Miro VI, Green M, Mazur L. Coomparison of different metronidazole therapeutic regiments for bacterial vaginosis. JAMA 1992; 268:92-95.

69. Glass G, McGaw B, Smith M. Meta-Analysis in Social Research. Newberry Park, CA, Sage Publications 1981:123-125, 218.

70. Oliver LD, Mehta R, Sarles HE. Acute renal failure following administration of ethylenediamine-tetraacetic acid (EDTA). Tex Med 1984; 80:40-42.

71. Dudley HR, Ritchie AC, Schilling A, Baker WH. Pathologic changes associated with the use of sodium ethylene diamine tetra-acetate in the treatment of hypercalcemia. N Engl J Med 1955; 252:331-337.

72. Cranton EM, Brecher A. Bypassing Bypass. New York, Stein and Day 1984.

73. Chappell LT, Kienow NT. The cost effectiveness of alternative medicine in the workplace. Chicago, Great Lakes Association of Clinical Medicine, Jack Hank, Executive Director, 70 West Huron Street, Chicago, IL 60610, 1993.

Appendix II

EDTA Chelation Treatment for Vascular Disease:
A Meta-Analysis Using Unpublished Data

by
L. Terry Chappell, M.D., John P. Stahl, Ph.D.,
and Ronald Evans, M.A.

Published in
Journal of Advancement in Medicine
Volume 7, Number 3, Fall 1994

ABSTRACT: The authors previously reported the results of a meta-analysis on the correlation between EDTA therapy and improvement in cardiovascular function where only published data were used in the analysis.[1] Many analysts suggest that using exclusively published data in a meta-analysis leads to a lowered confidence level in the results because of the possibility of publication bias. In order to improve the confidence level, if possible, in the results of their original paper, the authors repeated the study using unpublished data. Unpublished "file drawer" data were collected from 32 clinicians who utilize intravenous EDTA with essentially the same protocol as was used in the original study. Various objective measurements demonstrate improvement in 1086 or 88 percent of the 1241 patients reported with an overall correlation coefficient of 0.88. A comparison of the studies using unpublished data with published data shows that the results are essentially the same. These data provide additional confidence of the effectiveness of EDTA treatment.

Background

Intravenous EDTA with trace minerals and vitamins has

been used in conjunction with lifestyle changes to treat vascular disease by a growing number of physicians. The authors conducted a meta-analysis[1] that showed a high positive correlation between treatment with EDTA and improvement in vascular disease. Included in the meta-analysis were 18 published articles and one large study that had been submitted for publication. All of the studies included in the meta-analysis met the criteria that there were data on individual patients and that objective testing was utilized in measuring outcomes.

Of the 22,765 patients analyzed, 19,779 or 87 percent showed measurable improvement after treatment. The overall correlation coefficient was 0.88. A meaningful interpretation of a correlation coefficient using Rosenthal and Rubin's binomial effect size display[1] is that for a correlation coefficient of 0.88 we would expect an increase of success in cardiovascular improvement from 6 percent of patients improved with no treatment to 94 percent of patients improved as a result of applying EDTA chelation therapy. The original meta-analysis, as conducted, offered very strong evidence of the effectiveness of EDTA chelation therapy in the treatment of cardiovascular disease.

A Bias Criticism of Meta-Analysis

One of the criticisms of meta-analysis is that when only published data is used in the analysis, there is potential for a type I publication error to exist. A type I error is the rejection of the null hypothesis when it is in fact true. For our case, the null hypothesis is "EDTA chelation therapy does not improve cardiovascular function." The basic premise regarding this criticism of meta-analysis is that there is a tendency to publish only positive or significant results and that results that are not significant remain unpublished. This is sometimes called the "file drawer problem."[2] One of two approaches can be used when addressing the possibility of a type I publication error. Either estimate the number of additional studies with nonsignificant results needed to nullify the significant result of the published data, or acquire unpublished data and include or compare the unpublished results with the published results. If the two results are significantly different then the result of the original analysis is suspect and the difference between the two needs to be resolved.

Cook and associates[3] recently wrote about the importance of the inclusion of unpublished data when performing a meta-analysis, especially when evaluating controversial medical therapies. Additionally, Wolf[4] in his "Guidelines for Practice" recommends that those researchers conducting a meta-analysis "search for unpublished studies in order to test for a type I error publication bias." In order to address the question regarding the validity of the results of our original paper, i.e., the existence of a type I publishing error, the authors decided to search for unpublished data in order to make a comparison between published data results and unpublished data results. Additional unpublished data were solicited by asking members of the American College for Advancement in Medicine (ACAM) to submit unpublished data from their individual medical practices. This paper reports and analyzes the results of this effort.

Unpublished Data Limitation

There are several problems to consider in the search for unpublished data for inclusion in a meta-analysis. Two of the more serious problem areas are obtaining a representative data set and the acquisition of good data. An unpublished data set is representative when the data come from a sample of the population equivalent to the population of the original meta-analysis. Data are good where adequate control conditions exist. Control of data is adequate when existing threats to internal and external validity and reliability are minimized. Those who argue against the inclusion of unpublished data without peer review in an analysis typically indicate that peer review in the publication process is meant to protect the reader from substandard material or inadequate data. Peer review is used to insure that those papers included in the publication meet certain minimum standards. Bypassing the peer review process by using unpublished data allows for the possibility of erroneous conclusions to be made because of the introduction of substandard data.

Being cognizant of these dangers, the authors collected additional unpublished data from practitioners of EDTA chelation therapy. The advantage of using unpublished data from this source has the following benefits. The sample data set is selected from a population which approximates the sample from the population of the original meta-analysis. The integrity of the individual data sets across the different study sets with respect to both validity and reliability is high for the following reasons. The protocol used in EDTA chelation therapy has been standardized, although minor variations are allowed, and physicians who administer the EDTA treatment have all been trained and certified to use the protocol. For objective data collection, the test procedures, equipment used, and interpretation of results for EDTA chelation therapy are all standard in the general practice of medicine and are accepted by practitioners in the field. No obscure or unusual protocols are needed in the administration of EDTA chelation therapy.

Method of Data Acquisition and Reduction

Two letters of solicitation were written and three requests from the podium at national meetings were made to the membership of ACAM requesting unpublished data. Data type was limited to the results of treating vascular disease with EDTA chelation therapy. The criteria for data collection were as follows:

1. Consecutive patients with objective testing done before and after treatment were to be included.

2. All patients must have had vascular disease with such diagnoses as coronary artery disease, peripheral vascular disease and/or cerebral vascular disease specified.

3. Treatment given was required to be according to the published protocol[5] that all members agree to use. The protocol includes 20-30 treatments of intravenous EDTA with specified additives, oral nutritional supplements, and lifestyle changes as needed.

4. Well-accepted, objective testing was required to show whether each patient improved or not with treatment.

5. Published data were excluded.

The data were then tabulated. Correlation coefficients were calculated for each investigator and for the entire collection of unpublished data. For comparison purposes correlation coefficients were also included for only published data and for the entire collection including both published and unpublished data.

The correlation coefficients were calculated in the following manner. There are two variables considered in this analysis. The first is the method of treatment and the second is the degree of improvement. Additionally these two variables are conditioned to be discrete dichotomies. The method of treatment variable then is limited to the values, EDTA chelation therapy versus no therapy and the degree of improvement variable is limited to the values of significant cardiovascular improvement versus little or no improvement, or worse. Formulating the variables in this way allows for the calculation of the phi (-) coefficient, a special case of the Pearson r correlation coefficient when both variables are discrete dichotomies. After the phi (-) correlation coefficients are calculated for the individual studies, the overall result of the meta-analysis is determined. The composite - is a synthesis of the results of each of the individual studies. It is formulated by calculating a weighted average correlation coefficient where each individual study correlation used is weighted by the number of patients in the particular study. The details and assumptions of this method of data reduction were published.[1]

Results

As is shown in Table 1, 32 physicians provided data on 1241 patients, 1086 of whom (88 percent) had measurable improvements by objective testing. Even though the inclusion of the several studies consisting of "one" patient can be statistically criticized, we have chosen to include them to show the robustness of the therapy. We also note that the correlation coefficient is the same with and without the studies of "one" patient. The overall correlation coefficient between treatment with EDTA and improvement in vascular disease was 0.88, which is a high positive correlation. Table 2 shows the testing and results of each doctor who provided data. Table 3 indicates that for the collection of all studies, published and unpublished, the overall correlation coefficient is 0.88. Table 4, the original meta-analysis results, shows that the overall correlation coefficient for the set of published studies is also 0.88. Since the correlation coefficient of 0.88 is the same for both the published and unpublished data, we conclude that there is no type I publication error. Our trust in the statement that "there is significant cardiovascular improvement associated with the treatment of EDTA chelation therapy" is much stronger as a result of this follow up meta-analysis using unpublished data.

Discussion

The results of this collection of unpublished data correspond remarkably well with the meta-analysis of published and pre-publication studies. Both sets of data reflect a high correlation between improvement in cardiovascular function and treatment with EDTA. The largest published series to date was the 2870 patients reported by Olszewer and Carter.[6] All of these reports show that at least 87 percent of vascular patients show measurable improvement with EDTA treatment.

All of the 32 clinicians whose work is described in this paper used the ACAM protocol for treatment of various vascular diseases. As noted in Tables 3 and 4, most of the data sets contained lifestyle changes, but there were a few in the original meta-analysis which did not. Although the correlation coefficients in the no-lifestyle-change data sets were also high, the numbers were too small to draw additional conclusions. One of the contributors in the original meta-analysis and two in this unpublished group used a lesser dose of 1.5 grams of EDTA rather than the usual dose of 3 grams. It is beyond the scope of this paper to compare the two doses, but the subset correlation coefficients were essentially the same and this did not affect the overall results.

The tests performed by each physician varied, but they were similar and commonly accepted. There were also minor variations in the type of nutritional supplements used.

The results of this paper confirm the effectiveness of EDTA chelation therapy in the treatment of cardiovascular disease.

Acknowledgments

The authors extend their appreciation to the American College for Advancement in Medicine for a grant that partially supported the gathering of this data and also to Sara Bassitt, who helped process and organize it.

Table 1
Correlation Coefficient Data for Unpublished Studies
Overall Correlation Coefficient = 0.88

Author	Type Study	Subjects	Improved	Same/Worse	Correlation
Garg	B,D,F,H	32	31	1	0.97
Hart	B,D,F,H	7	7	0	1.00
Hodara	B,D,F,H	1	1	0	1.00
Janson	B,D,F,H	10	7	3	0.73
Laird	B,D,F,H	19	12	7	0.68
Affandi	B,D,F,H	10	10	0	1.00
Bock	B,D,F,H	11	10	1	0.91
Born	B,D,F,G	748	645	103	0.87
Darbro	B,D,F,H	10	10	0	1.00
Goldberg	B,D,F,H	4	3	1	0.77
Gonzalez	B,D,F,H	3	3	0	1.00
Gunter	B,D,F,H	7	6	1	0.87
Eckerly, Dole	B,D,F,H	19	19	0	1.00
Harris	B,D,F,H	1	1	0	1.00
Maulfair	B,D,F,H	9	8	1	0.89
Penwell	B,D,F,H	49	42	7	0.87
Reynoso	B,D,F,H	8	8	0	1.00
Chappell	B,D,F,H	33	27	6	0.83
Sams	B,D,F,H	18	18	0	1.00
Magaziner	B,D,F,H	1	1	0	1.00
Speckhart	B,D,F,H	1	1	0	1.00
Young	B,D,F,H	35	32	3	0.92
Braverman	B,D,F,H	1	1	0	1.00
Rozema	B,D,F,G	53	50	3	0.94
Kindness	B,D,F,H	29	26	3	0.90
DeSouza	B,D,F,H	9	9	0	1.00
Moharram	B,D,F,H	1	1	0	1.00
Olzsewer, et al	B,D,F,H	30	26	4	0.87
Godfrey	B,D,F,H	16	16	0	1.00
Levin	B,D,F,H	22	15	7	0.72
Wolverton	B,D,F,H	21	19	2	0.91
Walker	B,D,F,H	23	21	2	0.92
TOTALS		1241	1086	155	

Study types: A - No Lifestyle Changes; B - Lifestyle Changes; C - Published Data; D - Unpublished Data; E - Large Studies, F - Small Studies, G - 1.5 gm. dose, H - 3.0 gm. dose

Table 2
STUDIES USED IN META-ANALYSIS

AUTHOR	SOURCE/ DATE	DIAGNOSES	TEST	SUB-JECTS	IMPROVED	SAME or WORSE
Olszewer, Carter	M Hypoth/88	CAD, PVD, CVD	SEKG, Dplr, WD	2,482	2,379	103
Clarke	A J Med Sc/56	CAD	Exercise activ	20	19	1
Kitchell, et al	A J Card/63	Severe CAD	Ex Act/prolong life	38	23	15
Sloth-Nielson	A J Surg/92	PVD, Smokers	Arteriograms	30	2	28
Casdorph	J H Med/81	CVD	TECH99	15	14	1
Casdorph, Farr	J H Med/83	PVD/Gangrene	Avoid amputation	4	4	0
Casdorph	J H Med/81	ASHD	TECH99/EjFx	18	17	1
Olszewer, Carter	J H Med As/91	PVD	A/B index, W Dist	10	10	0
Godfrey	NZMJ/90	PVD	Doppler, A/B index	27	25	2
Morgan	J Adv Med/91	CAD	Stress EKG	2	2	0
Bruck-nerova	Cas Lekces/80	PVD	WD, arteriograms	2	2	0
Hancke	-/93	CAD, PVD	Avoid bypass/amput	92	82	10
Hancke	-/93	CAD	SEKG/STseg	253	175	78
Hancke	-/93	PVD	(A/B Index), W Dist	(262) 308	(217) 272	(45) 36
McGillem	NEJM/88	CAD, Renal Dis.	Angiograms	1	0	1
Rudolph, McDonagh	J Adv Med/90	CVD	Doppler/Ultrasound	1	1	0
McDonagh, et al	J Adv Med/82	CVD	Ocu CV Analysis	57	50	7
McDonagh, et al	J Adv Med/85	PVD	A/B Syst BP	117	95	22
Hoekstra, et al	-/93	PVD, CVD	Thermography	19,147	16,466	2,681
Van der Schaar	J Adv Med/89	CAD, CVD, PVD	Exercise Tolerance	111	111	0
Rudolph, et al	J Adv Med/91	CVD	Carotid Ultrasound	30	30	0
TOTAL-19 STUDIES				22,765	19,779 (87%)	2986 (13%)

Table 3
Correlation Coefficient Data for Unpublished Studies
Overall Correlation Coefficient = 0.88 "All Data"

Author	Type Study	Subjects	Improved	Same/Worse	Correlation
Olszewer, Carter	B,C,E,H	2482	2379	103	0.96
Clarke	A,C,F,H	20	19	1	0.95
Kitchell, et al	A,C,F,H	38	23	15	0.66
Sloth-Nielson	B,C,F,H	30	2	28	0.19
Casdorph	B,C,F,H	15	14	1	0.94
Casdorph, Farr	B,C,F,H	4	4	0	1.00
Casdorph	B,C,F,H	18	17	1	0.95
Olszewer, Carter	A,C,F,G	10	10	0	1.00
Godfrey	B,C,F,H	27	25	2	0.93
Morgan	B,C,F,H	2	2	0	1.00
Bru.cknerova	A,C,F,H	2	2	0	1.00
Hancke	B,C,F,H	92	82	10	0.90
Hancke	B,C,F,H	253	175	78	0.73
Hancke	B,C,F,H	308	272	36	0.89
McGillem	B,C,F,H	1	0	1	0.00
Rudolph, McDonagh	B,C,F,H	1	1	0	1.00
McDonagh, et al	B,C,F,H	57	50	7	0.88
McDonagh, et al	B,C,F,H	117	95	22	0.83
Hoekstra, et al	B.D.E.H	19147	16466	2681	0.87
Van der Schaar	B,C,F,H	111	111	0	1.00
Rudolph, et al	B,C,F,H	30	30	0	1.00
Garg	B,D,F,H	32	31	1	0.97
Hart	B,D,F,H	7	7	0	1.00
Hodara	B,D,F,H	1	1	0	1.00
Janson	B,D,F,H	10	7	3	0.73
Laird	B,D,F,H	19	12	7	0.68
Affandi	B,D,F,H	10	10	0	1.00
Bok	B,D,F,H	11	10	1	0.91
Born	B,D,F,G	748	645	103	0.87
Darbro	B,D,F,H	10	10	0	1.00
Goldberg	B,D,F,H	4	3	1	0.77
Gonzalez	B,D,F,H	3	3	0	1.00
Gunter	B,D,F,H	7	6	1	0.87
2Eckerly, Dole	B,D,F,H	19	19	0	1.00
Harris	B,D,F,H	1	1	0	1.00
Maulfair	B,D,F,H	9	8	1	0.89
Penwell	B,D,F,H	49	42	7	0.87
Reynoso	B,D,F,H	8	8	0	1.00
Chappell	B,D,F,H	33	27	6	0.83
Sams	B,D,F,H	18	18	0	1.00
Magaziner	B,D,F,H	1	1	0	1.00
Speckhart	B,D,F,H	1	1	0	1.00
Young	B,D,F,H	35	32	3	0.92
Braverman	B,D,F,H	1	1	0	1.00
Rozema	B,D,F,G	53	50	3	0.94
Kindness	B,D,F,H	29	26	3	0.90
DeSouza	B,D,F,H	9	9	0	1.00
Moharran	B,D,F,H	1	1	0	1.00
Olszewer, et al	B,D,F,H	30	26	4	0.87
Godfrey	B,D,F,H	16	16	0	1.00
Levin	B,D,F,H	22	15	7	0.72
Wolverton	B,D,F,H	21	19	2	0.91
H. Walker	B,D,F,H	23	21	2	0.92
Totals		**24006**	**20865**	**3141**	

Study types: A - No Lifestyle Changes; B - Lifestyle Changes; C - Published Data; D - Unpublished Data; E - Large Studies, F - Small Studies, G - 1.5 gm. dose, H - 3.0 gm. dose

Table 4
Correlation Coefficient Data for Unpublished Studies
Overall Correlation Coefficient = 0.88

Author	Type Study	Sub-jects	Improved	Same/ Worse	Correla-tion
Olszewer, Carter	B,C,E,H	2482	2379	103	0.96
Clarke	A,C,F,H	20	19	1	0.95
Kitchell, et al	A,C,F,H	38	23	15	0.66
Sloth-Nielson	B,C,F,H	30	2	28	0.19
Casdorph	B,C,F,H	15	14	1	0.94
Casdorph, Farr	B,C,F,H	4	4	0	1.00
Casdorph	B,C,F,H	18	17	1	0.95
Olszewer, Carter	A,C,F,G	10	10	0	1.00
Godfrey	B,C,F,H	27	25	2	0.93
Morgan	B,C,F,H	2	2	0	1.00
Brucknerova	A,C,F,H	2	2	0	1.00
Hancke	B,C,F,H	92	82	10	0.90
Hancke	B,C,F,H	253	175	78	0.73
Hancke	B,C,F,H	308	272	36	0.89
McGillem	B,C,F,H	1	0	1	0.00
Rudolph, McDonagh	B,C,F,H	1	1	0	1.00
McDonagh, et al	B,C,F,H	57	50	7	0.88
McDonagh, et al	B,C,F,H	117	95	22	0.83
Hoekstra, et al	B,D,E,H	19147	16466	2681	0.87
Van der Schaar	B,C,F,H	111	111	0	1.00
Rudolph, et al	B,C,F,H	30	30	0	1.00

Study types: A - No Lifestyle Changes; B - Lifestyle Changes; C - Published Data; D - Unpublished Data; E - Large Studies, F - Small Studies, G - 1.5 gm. dose, H - 3.0 gm. dose

References

1. Chappell LT, Stahl JP. The correlation between EDTA chelation therapy and improvement in cardiovascular function: a meta-analysis. J Adv Med 1993; 6: 139-160.

2. Rosenthal R. The "File Drawer Problem" and tolerance for null results. Psychological Bulletin 1979; 86: 638-641.

3. Cook DJ, Guyatt GH, Ryan G, et al. Should unpublished data be included in meta-analyses? JAMA 1993; 269: 2749- 2753.

4. Wolf FM. Meta-analysis: Quantitative Methods for Research Synthesis. Newberry Park, CA. Sage Publications 1986:55.

5. Cranton EM. Protocol of American College of Advancement in Medicine for the safe and effective administration of EDTA chelation therapy. J Adv Med 1989; 2:269-306.

6. Olszewer E, Carter JP. EDTA chelation therapy in chronic degenerative disease. Med Hypoth 1988; 27:41-49.

Appendix III

References for Julian Whitaker's Preface
on the Misuse of Bypass Surgery and Angioplasty

Parisi AF, Folland ED, Hartigan PA. Comparison of angioplasty with medical therapy in the treatment of single-vessel coronary artery disease. New England Journal of Medicine 1992; 326: 1.

The Associated Press, Angioplasty Supported over Drugs in Report. Researchers find better recovery with use of heart surgery. Jan 2, 1992.

Ornish D, Scherwitz LW, et al. The Effects of Stress Management Training and Dietary Changes in Treating Ischemic Heart Disease. JAMA 1983; 249: 54-59.

Ornish D, Brown SE. Can Lifestyle Changes Reverse Coronary Heart Disease? The Lancet 1990; 366: 129.

Statistics supplied by the Institute for Health Policy Studies, University of California at San Francisco, based upon hospital discharge data from the Office of Statewide Health Planning and Development.

Aleshire P. Rise in angioplasties labeled "major problem." "Willy nilly" use to clear arteries "business-driven." The Arizona Republic Nov 19, 1989. Discharge Data/Summarization Data from Health Care Financing Administration on 1,030 angioplasties.

Hartzler GO. The learning curve in coronary angioplasty. Cardiology 1988; 5: 3.

Braunwald E. Coronary-artery surgery at the crossroads. New England Journal of Medicine 1977; 297: 661-663.

Dougherty E, Hagin D. The future looks bright for cardiac catheterization. Health Care Strategic Management, the newsletter for hospital strategists 1989; 7: 1.

Graboys T. Conflicts of interest in the management of silent ischemia. JAMA 1989; 261: 2116-2117.

Council on Scientific Affairs and Council on Ethical and Judicial Affairs, Conflicts of Interest in medical center industry research relationships. JAMA 1990; 263: 2790.

Palca J. NIH grapples with conflict of interest. Science 1989; 245: 23.

Blumenthal D. University industry research relationships in biotechnology implications for the university. Science 1986; 232: 1361-1366.

Webster's Third New International Dictionary

Shulkin DJ. Choice of specialty: It's money that matters in the USA. JAMA 262: 1630.

CASS Principal Investigators and the Associates: Coronary artery Surgery Study (CASS): A randomized trial of coronary artery bypass surgery: Survival data. Circulation 1983; 68: 939-950.

Podrid PJ, Graboys TB, Lown B. Prognosis of medically treated patients with coronary-artery disease with profound ST-segment depression during exercise testing. New England Journal of Medicine 1981; 305: 1111-1116.

Graboys TB, et al. Results of a second-opinion program for coronary artery bypass grafting surgery. JAMA 1987; 258: 1611-1614.

Graboys TB, Biegelsen B, Lampert S, Blatt CM, Lown B. Results of a second-opinion trial among patients recommended for coronary angiography. JAMA 1992; 258: 2537-2540.

McIntosh HD, Garcia JD. The first decade of aortocoronary bypass grafting, 1967-1977: A review. Circulation 1975; 57: 405-531.

Braunwald E. Editorial Retrospective. Effects of coronary-artery bypass grafting on survival; Implications of the randomized coronary-artery surgery study. An editorial. The New England Journal of Medicine 1983; 309: 1181-1184.

McIntosh HD. Second opinions for aortocoronary bypass grafting are beneficial. JAMA 1987; 258: 1644-1645.

Hueb W, Bellotti G, Ramirez J, et al. Two-to-eight-year survival rates in patients who refused coronary artery bypass grafting. The American Journal of Cardiology 1989; 63: 155-159.

Whitaker, JM. The angioplasty enthusiasm without proof. Reversing Heart Disease. Warner Books 1985.

White CW, Wright CB, Doty DB, Hiratza L, Eastham CL, Harrison DG, Marcus ML. Does Visual Interpretation of the Coronary Arteriogram Predict the Physiologic Importance of a Coronary Stenosis? From the Cardiovascular Division, Department of Internal Medicine and the Section of Cardiothoracic Surgery, Department of Surgery, University of Iowa Hospitals and Veterans Administration Hospital, Iowa City, IA.

Zir LM, Miller SW, Dinsmore RE, Gilbert JP, Harthorne JW. Interobserver variability in coronary angiography. Circulation 1976; 53: 627-32.

DeRouen TA, Murray JA, Owen W. Variability in the analysis of coronary arteriograms. Circulation 1977; 55: 324-8.

Sellman M, Ivert T, Wahlgren NG, Knutsson E, Semb BK. Early neurological and electroencephalographic changes after coronary artery surgery in low-risk patients younger than 70 years. Thoracic and Cardiovascular Surgeon 1991; 51: 443-7.

Slogoff S, Reul GJ, Keats AS, Curry GR, Crum ME, Elmquist BA, Giesecke NM, Jistel JR, Rogers LK, Soderberg JD, et al. Role of perfusion pressure and flow in major organ dysfunction after cardiopulmonary bypass. Annals of Thoracic Surgery 1990; 50: 911-8.

Arom KV, Cohen DE, Strobl FT. Effect of intraoperative intervention on neurological outcome based on electroencephalographic monitoring during cardiopulmonary bypass. Annals of Thoracic Surgery 1988; 48: 476-83.

Deverall PB, Padayachee TS, Parsons S, Theobold R, Battistessa SA. Ultrasound detection of micro-emboli in the middle cerebral artery during cardiopulmonary bypass surgery. European Journal of Cardio-Thoracic Surgery 1988; 4: 256-60.

Nevin M, Colchester AC, Adams S, Pepper JR. Evidence for involvement of hypocapnia and hypoperfusion in aetiology of neurological deficit after cardiopulmonary bypass. Lancet 1987; 2: 1493-5.

Cashin WL, Sanmarco ME, Nessim SA, Blankenhorn DH. Accelerated progression of atherosclerosis in coronary vessels with minimal lesions that are bypassed. New England Journal of Medicine 1984; 311: 824-828.

Wiseman A, Waters DD, Walling A, Pelletier GB, Roy D, Theroux P. Long-term prognosis after myocardial infarction in patients with previous coronary artery bypass surgery. J Am Coll Cardiol 1988; 12: 873-880.

Edmunds LH, Stephenson LW, Edie RN, Ratcliffe MB. Open-heart surgery in octogenarians. New England Journal of Medicine 1988; 319: 131-136.

Appendix IV

I. Removal of iron, copper, aluminum and heavy metals. Has antioxidant effect in quenching free radicals.

A. Cranton EM, Frackelton JP: Free radical pathology in age-associated diseases: treatment with EDTA chelation, nutrition and antioxidants. J Hol Med 1984; 6: 6-37.

ABSTRACT: Recent discoveries in the field of free radical pathology provide a coherent, unifying scientific basis to explain many of the diverse benefits reported from treatment with EDTA Chelation Therapy. The free radical concept provides a scientific basis for treatment and prevention of the major causes of disability and death; including atherosclerosis, dementia, cancer, arthritis and numerous other diseases. EDTA Chelation Therapy, hyperbaric oxygen therapy, applied clinical nutrition, nutritional supplementation, physical exercise and moderation of health destroying habits all have common therapeutic mechanisms which reduced free radical causes of many age-associated diseases.

B. Gutteridge, JMC: Ferrous-salt-promoted damage to deoxyribose and benzoate, the increased effectiveness of hydroxyl-radical scavengers in the presence of EDTA. Biochem J 1987; 243: 709-714.

ABSTRACT: Hydroxyl radicals (OH^{-1}) in free solution react with scavengers at rates predictable from their known second-order rate constants. However, when OH^{-1} radicals are produced in biological systems by metal-ion-dependent Fenton-type reactions scavengers do not always appear to conform to these established rate *constants. The detector molecules deoxyribose and benzoate were used to study damage by OH^{-1} involving a hydrogen-abstraction reaction and an aromatic hydroxylation. In the presence of EDTA the rate constant for the reaction of scavengers with OH^{-1} was generally higher than in the absence of EDTA. This radiomimetic effect of EDTA can be explained by the removal of iron from the detector molecule, where it brings about a site-specific reaction, by EDTA allowing more OH^{-1} radicals to escape into free solution to react with added scavengers. The deoxyribose assay, although chemically complex, in the presence of EDTA appears to give a simple and cheap method of obtaining rate constants for OH^{-1} reactions that compare well with these obtained by using pulse radiolysis.*

C. Deucher DP: EDTA Chelation Therapy: an antioxidant strategy. J Advancement in Med 1988; 1: 182-190.

ABSTRACT: A new understanding of many degenerative diseases of aging is proposed, based on recent findings in the areas of molecular biology and oxygen free radical reactions. EDTA Chelation Therapy causes an increased excretion of polyvalent metals from the body, both toxic heavy metals and transition metals which catalyze free radical pathology. Antioxidant effects are proposed as a cause of the observed clinical benefits following intravenous EDTA Chelation Therapy.

D. Bjorksten J: Possibilities and limitations of chelation as a means for life extension. J Adv in Med 1989; 2: 77-78.

ABSTRACT: An overview is presented of functions and limitations of chelation for removing undesired metals, including but not limited to acute poisons, chronic environmental poisons, bone-seeking radioisotopes, and cumulative poisons active in senile dementias and scleroses. The chelating techniques are applicable to all metals. Present trends include the development of injectable or oral chelation. Among promising developments are mentioned cholyl hydroxamic acid, which discharges metal through the liver and digestive tract as well as by the diney route, and other orally administrable chelators which on the basis of animal tests appear to have advantages over those now in use.

E. Zylke J: Studying oxygen's life-and-death roles if taken from or reintroduced into tissue. JAMA 1988; 259: 964-5.

F. Lamb DJ, Leake DS: The effect of EDTA on the oxidation of low density lipoprotein. Atherosclerosis 1992; 94: 35-42.

ABSTRACT: Low density lipoprotein (LDL) is routinely isolated and stored in buffers containing ethylenediamine-tetra-acetic acid (EDTA) to inhibit its autoxidation. We have investigated the effect of EDTA on LDL oxidation by both copper ions and macrophages. LDL oxidation by macrophages in Ham's F-10 medium containing 6 uM iron showed a large and concentration-dependent increase when EDTA was added up to about 10 uM. EDTA concentrations above about 10 uM progressively inhibited LDL oxidation as measured by macrophage degradation, thiobarbituric acid-reactive substances and electrophoretic mobility. The oxidation of LDL by 1 uM copper in Ham's F-10 medium, measured by macrophage degradation, also show a large increase with low concentrations of EDTA (1-3 uM), with higher concentrations (10 uM or above) strongly inhibiting the oxidation. In a simple phosphate buffer, however, EDTA simply inhibited the oxidation of LDL by copper with equimolar amounts of EDTA to copper giving a complete inhibition. The results of this study indicate that when LDL oxidation by cells or by copper in Ham's F-10 medium is investigated, more oxidation may be obtained if the EDTA is not previously removed from the LDL preparation.

G. Rahko PS, Salerni R, Uretsky BF: Successful reversal by Chelation Therapy of congestive cardiomyopathy due to iron overload. J Am Coll Card 1986; 8: 436-40.

ABSTRACT: A patient who developed severe iron overload cardiomyopathy is described. Venesection could not be performed because the patient had chronic anemia. Deferoxamine mesylate, a chelating agent, was administered daily for more than 2 years and produced significant improvement in ventricular function which was associated with a biopsy-proven decrease in myocardial iron stores. This is the first reported case in which a severe cardiomyopathy due to iron overload was reversed by Chelation Therapy alone.

H. DeBoer DA, Clark RE: Iron chelation in myocardial preservation after ischemia-reperfusion injury: The importance of pretreatment and toxicity. Ann Thorac Surg 1992; 53: 412-8.

I. Menasche P, Pinwica A: Free radicals and myocardial protection: a surgical viewpoint. Ann Thorac Surg 1989; 47: 939-45.

J. Link G, Pinson A, Hershko C: Heart cells in culture: a model of myocardial iron overload and chelation. J Lab Clin Med 1985; 106: 147-53.

K. Freeman AP, Giles RW, Berdoukas VA, Walsh WR, Choy D, Murray PC: Early left ventricular dysfunction and Chelation Therapy in thalassemia major. Ann Intern Med 1983; 99: 450-4.

L. Halstead BM: The Scientific Basis of EDTA Chelation Therapy, Colton, California, Golden Quill Publishers 1979.

M. Rudolph CJ, McDonagh EW, Barber RK: Effect of EDTA chelation on serum iron. J Adv in Med 1991; 4: 39-45.
    ABSTRACT: One hundred and twenty-two patients suffering from various chronic degenerative disorders were evaluated objectively for fasting serum iron values before and after EDTA (ethylenediamine tetracetic acid) chelation plus multivitamin mineral (excluding iron) supplementation. After 30 intravenous 3 gram treatments of EDTA, average serum iron levels dropped 17.5% (t-4.230, P). Abnormally high initial iron decreased 43.1% (t=7.602, p), while low initial iron increased 41% (t=3.30, p).

II. Removal of Metastatic Calcium

A. Kaman RL, Rudolph CJ, McDonagh EW, Walker FM: Effect of EDTA Chelation Therapy on aortic calcium in rabbits on atherogenic diets: quantitative and histochemical studies. J Adv in Med 1990; 3: 13-22.

ABSTRACT: A group of rabbits were sub-divided into two subgroups, the first being placed on a standard laboratory diet while the second was placed on a high cholesterol containing atherogenic diet. The animals were either infused with EDTA, saline or nothing (in the controls) followed by sacrificing and the aortas were examined for calcium both microscopically, using calcium stains, and quantitatively. Results indicated significantly less calcium in the aortas of the EDTA infused animals when compared to both controls and saline infused animals.

B. Levy RJ, Howard SL, Oshry LJ: Carboxyglutamic acid (Gla) containing proteins of human calcified atherosclerotic plaque solubilized by EDTA. Molecular weight distribution and relationship to osteocalcin. Atherosclerosis 1986; 59: 155-60.

ABSTRACT: Proteins containing the calcium binding amino acid, gamma-carboxyglutamic acid (Gla), are abundant in calcified human atherosclerotic plaque, but are detectable only at trace levels in the normal arterial wall and non-mineralized atherosclerotic lesions. These proteins have been incompletely characterized, and their role in the pathophysiology of atherosclerosis is not known. The present study sought to determine the overall molecular weight distribution of the calcified plaque Gla-protein fraction solubilized by EDTA demineralization and the possible relationship of these proteins to the bone Gla-protein, osteocalcin. Calcified atheromata were demineralized with EDTA (0.5 M, pH 6.9) for 7 days and the dialyzed EDTA extract subjected to procedures with tritium. The EDTA solubilized Gla-protein fraction (19.5% of the total Gla) was separated by gel filtration high performance liquid chromatography which demonstrated a single broad radiolabeled Gla-protein peak with an approximate molecular weight of 6000 daltons. In addition the EDTA solubilized atherosclerotic Gla-proteins could be distinguished from the bone Gla-protein, osteocalcin (molecular weight = 5700 daltons), by reverse phase HPLC and specific radioimmunoassays for os-

teocalcin. It is plaque solubilized with EDTA demineralization consist of a heterogeneous 6000 dalton fraction, which is apparently unrelated to the bone Gla-protein, osteocalcin.

C. Mallette LE, Hollis BW, Dunn K, Stinson M, Dunn JK, Wittels E, Gotto AM: Medical Service, Veterans Administration Medical Center, 2002 Holcombe Boulevard, Houston, TX 77030 USA. Ten weeks of intermittent hypocalcemic stimulation does not produce functional parathyroid hyperplasia. Am J Med Sci, 1991; 302: 138-141.

ABSTRACT: *Hypocalcemia is a major stimulus for parathyroid hormone secretion and presumably the major cause of parathyroid hyperplasia in chronic hypocalcemic syndromes. We could find no data to indicate what degree, duration, or frequency of hypocalcemia is needed to produce parathyroid hyperplasia in humans. We have monitored the effects of thrice weekly hypocalcemic parathyroid stimulation for 10 weeks. Measurements were made during a study designed to test the feasibility of carrying out a randomized, blinded trial of "Chelation Therapy," a widely used but unproven method to treat atherosclerotic symptoms. Eight patients received infusions of disodium ethylenediaminetetraacetic acid (EDTA) and six received placebo infusions thrice weekly for ten weeks. The EDTA (50 mg/hg over three hours) lowered serum ionized calcium at two hours by an average of 0.20 mmol/L and trebled the immunoreactive parathyroid hormone (iPTH) value. Basal serum iPTH, ionized calcium and 1,25-dihydroxyvitamin D values, measured just before the infusion, did not change significantly after 10 weeks of treatment with either EDTA or placebo. The increment in serum iPTH produced by the EDTA-induced hypocalcemia was also unchanged. Lowering ionized serum calcium to values below the normal range three times a week for 10 weeks is not a sufficient stimulus to cause a detectable increase in basal or stimulated parathyroid function.*

D. Walker FM, Wilson CW III, Kaman RL: Dept. Biol., NTSU/TCOM, Denton, Tex. 76203 USA. The effects of EDTA

Chelation Therapy on plaque calcium and plasma lipoproteins in atherosclerotic rabbits. Fed Proc 1979; 38 (No. 4335).

E. Walker F, Wilson C III, Kaman RL: North Texas State Univ., Texas Coll Osteopath. Med., Denton, Tex. USA. The effects of EDTA Chelation Therapy on plaque composition and serum lipoproteins in atherosclerotic rabbits. J Am Ost Assoc, 1978, 78: 144.

III. Anticoagulant Effects

A. Kindness G, Frackelton JP: Effect of ethylene diamine tetraacetic acid (EDTA) on platelet aggregation in human blood. J Adv in Med 1989; 2: 519-30.

ABSTRACT: Clinical administration of Ethylene Diamine Tetraacetic Acid (Na_2-EDTA) was examined with respect to the ex vivo aggregation of human blood platelets. The EDTA is shown to inhibit the aggregation of human blood platelets under certain conditions. Inhibition is noted on adenosine(ADP), epinephrine and thrombin-induced aggregation respectively. It is without effect on collagen-induced aggregation. These results are discussed in relation to the potential clinical effects exerted on platelets by EDTA and its possible role in hemostatic events.

B. Zurcker MB, Grant RA: Nonreversible loss of platelet aggregability induced by calcium deprivation. Blood 1978; 52: 505-13.

C. Lanza F, Stierle A, Gachet C, Cazenave JP: Differential effects of extra- and intracellular calcium chelation on human platelet function and glycoprotein-IIB-IIIA complex stability. Nouvelle Revue Francaise D Hematologie 1992; 34: 123-131.

D. Badimon L, Badimon JJ, Lassila R, Heras M, and other: Thrombin regulation of platelet interaction with damaged vessel wall and isolated collagen type-I at arterial flow conditions in a procine model—effects of hirudins, heparin and calcium chelation. Blood 1991; 78: 423-434.

E. May J, Loesche W, Heptinstall S: Glucose increases spontaneous platelet aggregation in whole blood. Journal: Throm Res 1990; 59: 489-495.

F. Perizzolo KE, Sullivan S, Waugh DF: Effects of calcium binding and of EDTA and CaEDTA on the clotting of bovine fibrinogen by thrombin. Arch Biochem Biophys 1985; 237: 520-534.

G. Suvorov AV, Markosyan RA: Some mechanisms of EDTA effect on platelet aggregation. Byull Eksp Biol Med 1981; 91: 587-590.

H. Zechmeister A, Malinovska V, Hadasova E, et al. Effect of glucagon on lipid and calcium deposition in arterial wall. Folla Morphol 1979: 27: 23-26.

I. Zechmeister A, Gulda O. Subcellular metabolism of CA2+ in smooth muscle and myocardium (an ultrahistochemical study). Folla Morphol 1981; 29: 333-335.

J. Malinovska V, Zechmeister A, Malinovska L., et al. The therapeutic effects of glucagon and chelation III on the arterial wall after experimental lipidosis and calcification. Scripta Medica 1983; 56: 391-400.

IV. Cell Membrane and Other Effects

A. Marban E, Koretsune Y, Corretti M, Chacko VP, Kusuka H: Calcium and its role in myocardial cell injury during ischemia and reperfusion. Circulation 1989; 80: 17-22.

B. Juneja S, Wolf M, McLennan R: Clumping of lymphoma cells in peripheral blood induced by EDTA. J Clin Pathol 1992; 45: 538-40.

C. Uhl HS, Dysko RC, St. Clair, RW: EDTA reduces liver cholesterol content in cholesterol-fed rabbits. Atherosclerosis 1992; 96: 181-8.

D. Kaman RL, Rudolph CJ, Galewaler J: Mineral excretion patterns during EDTA Chelation Therapy. J Amer Osteo Assoc 1977; 76: 471.

E. Gordon GB, Vance RB: EDTA Chelation Therapy for atherosclerosis: history and mechanisms of action. Ost Ann 1976; 4: 38-62.

F. Simon VC, Cohen RA: EDTA influences reactivity of isolated aorta from hypercholesterolemic rabbits. Am J Heart Circ Physiol 1992; 262: 31-5.

G. Busch L, Tessler J, Bazerque PM: Effects of calcium and EDTA on rat skin capillary permeability and on its response to histamine, serotonin, and bradykinin. Acta Physiol Pharmacol Latinoam (Argentina) 1989; 39: 227-234.

H. Valles J, Martinez-Sales V, Aznar J, Santos MT: The effect of EDTA on the production of prostacyclin by rat aorta. Thromb Res 1986; 43: 479-483.

I. Peng CF, Kame JJ, Bissett JK, et al: Improvement of oxidative phosphorylation by EDTA in mitochondria from acutely ischemic myocardium which has been reperfused. Clin Res 1977; 25: 244.

J. Altura BM, Altura BT: Magnesium withdrawal and contraction of arterial smooth muscle: effects of EDTA, EGTA, and divalent cations. Proc Soc Exp Biol Med 1976; 151: 752-755.

K. Solti F, Juhasz-Nagy S, Kecskemeti V, Czako B, Nemeth V, Kekesi V: Effect of the Ca2+ chelators EDTA and EGTA on sinoatrial-node activity and heart irritability. Acta Physiol Acad Sci Hung 1982; 60: 155-64.

L. Cranton EM, Frackelton JP: Current status of EDTA Chelation Therapy on occlusive arterial disease. J of Adv in Med 1989; 2: 107-119.

ABSTRACT: Benefits of intravenous Chelation Ther-

apy are unknown to most physicians. A series of circumstances led to the cessation of investigations and the lack of acceptance of an effective non-invasive therapy, which is less expensive and safer than by-pass surgery. This article addresses those circumstances. This review supports the use of EDTA Chelation Therapy in treatment of occlusive arterial disease and is a companion reference to reports of a series of recent, highly significant controlled studies showing the safety and effectiveness of this therapy.

M. Hagen PO, Davies MG, Schuman RW, Murray JJ: Reduction of vein graft intimal hyperplasia by ex vivo treatment with Desferrioxamine Manganese. J of Vasc Res 1992; 29: 405-409.

ABSTRACT: Reversed vein grafting exposes the venous tissue to a period of ischemia, reperfusion and subsequent free radical generation which may contribute to endothelial injury and/or damage, smooth muscle cell proliferation and the later development of intimal hyperplasia. The effects of ex vivo treatment with desferrioxamine Mn^{+3} (DFMn), a cell-permeable free radical scavenger, on the development of intimal hyperplasia in experimental vein grafts was examined. Twenty New Zealand white rabbits received a reversed vein interposition bypass graft into the ipsilateral common carotid artery. Ten explanted veins were immersed in a heparinized (5IU/ml) saline solution, and 10 others were immersed in a similar solution containing DFMn (1mM) for 45 minutes prior to reimplantation. There were no short-term functional or morphologic toxic side effects associated with DFMn treatment on either the endothelial or smooth muscle cells of the veins. At 28 days, grafts (n=20) were perfusion-fixed in vivo for histological and morphometric studies. There was a significant reduction in intimal thickening in the DFMn-treated group compared to the untreated group. The thicknesses of the intimal hyperplasia in the proximal segments were 50.6 6.3 vs. 76.9 3.2 %m (p 0.05), in the middle segments 42.0 5.0 vs. 88.3 6.2 %m (p 0.05) and in the distal segments 55.7 5.0 vs. 88.3 6.2 %m (p 0.05) for treated and untreated animals, respectively. No evidence of long-term toxicity was found.

These results indicate that a single ex vivo treatment with DFMn reduces graft intimal hyperplasia normally present at 4 weeks and suggests that oxygen free radicals may play a role in the initiation of vein graft intimal hyperplasia.

L. Terry Chappell, M.D., is in private practice in Bluffton, Ohio. He is President of the American College for Advancement of Medicine and is Assistant Professor of Family Practice at Wright State School of Medicine. Correspondence may be addressed to Dr. Chappell at:

The Celebration of Health Center
122 Thurman Street
Bluffton, OH 45817

Resources for those seeking doctors who give chelation:

Great Lakes Association of Clinical Medicine
1407-B North Wells Street
Chicago, IL 60610
800-286-6013

American College for Advancement in Medicine
23121 Verdugo Drive
Laguna Hills, CA 92653
800-532-3688